ENT TZAR

A Companion to DO-HNS and MRCS (ENT) OSCE Guide

Revision Questions with Answers

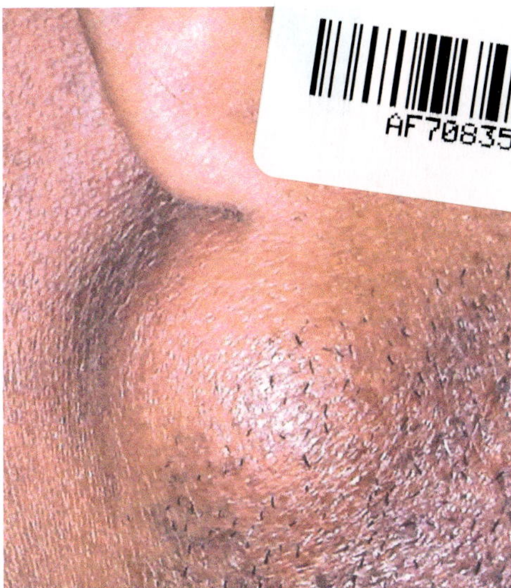

Ricardo A P Persaud

Adam C Gaunt | Konstantinos Argiris

1st Edition 2014

FastPrint Publishing

www.fast-print.net/store.php

A Companion to DO-HNS and MRCS (ENT) OSCE Guide: Revision Questions with Answers

A catalogue record for this book is available from the British Library

ISBN 978-178456-153-6

First published 2014 by
FASTPRINT PUBLISHING
Peterborough, England.

RICARDO A P PERSAUD
FRCS ORL-HNS (Eng) | CCT Otol (UK)
MB BS | MSB | CBiol | MPhil | MRCS (Gen) | DO-HNS
Consultant ENT Head Neck and Rhinoplastic Surgeon
Al Zahra Medical Group, Sharjah/Dubai, PO Box 3499, UAE.

ADAM C GAUNT
BA (Hons) | BM BS | MRCS (ENT)
Core Surgical Trainee, East of England Deanery, UK.

KONSTANTINOS ARGIRIS
BA (Hons) | BM BS | MRCS (ENT)
Specialty Registrar, KSS Deanery, UK.

Contents

Chapter 5 Imaging

Chapter 6 Manned Station Scenarios

Acknowledgement

Many thanks to Mr Owen Judd, Consultant ENT Surgeon, for his excellent editoral assistance.

Other publications by the ENTTZAR TEAM

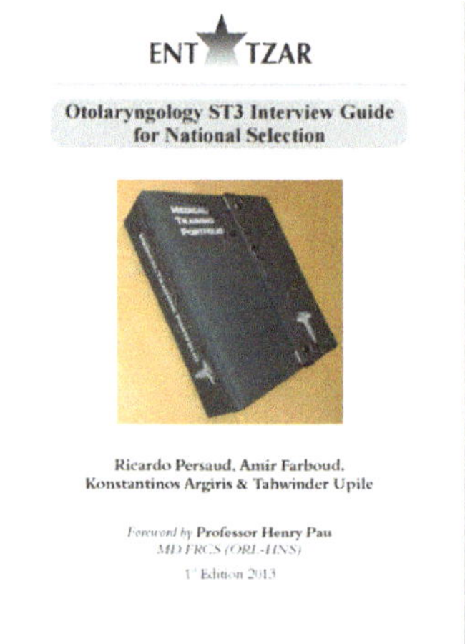

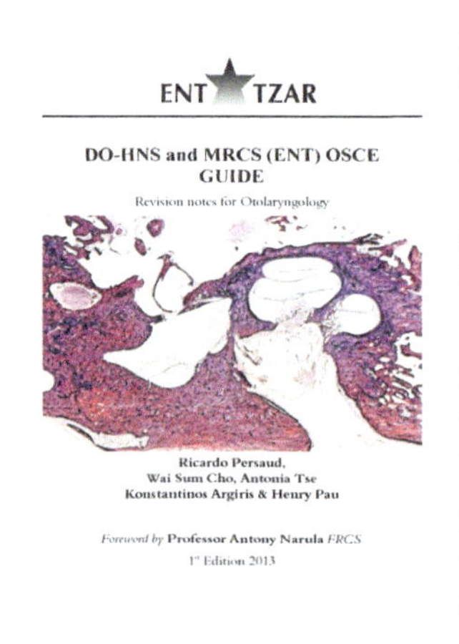

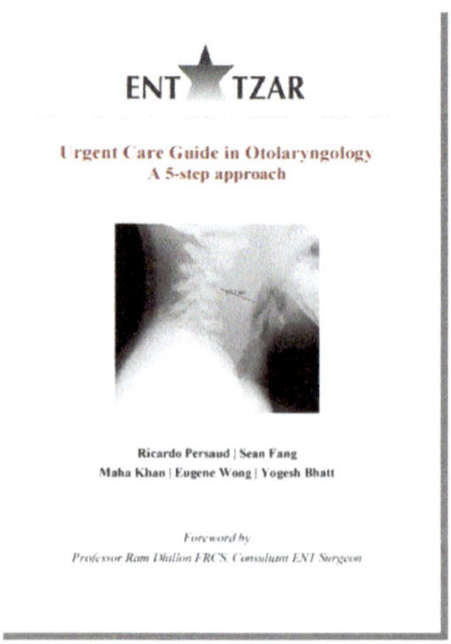

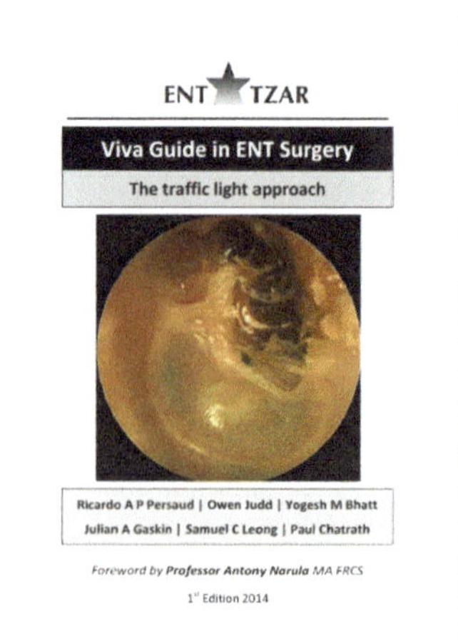

CHAPTER 1

Paediatric ENT

1.1 Nasal obstruction in a neonate

You are called to review a new-born baby who appears blue shortly after delivery but rapidly becomes pink on crying.

Questions

a) What is the most likely diagnosis and give 2 additional differential diagnoses?

b) Name two simple tests that may support your primary diagnosis?

c) What imaging is helpful in this condition?

d) Explain the embryological basis of this anomaly

e) What syndrome is associated with this condition and list 6 features of this syndrome.

f) What are the main surgical approaches to treat this newborn? List 2 only.

Answers

a) Bilateral choanal atresia. Differentials include (1) piriform aperture stenosis, (2) severe neonatal rhinitis (3) nasal masses such as glioma, encephalocele, meningoencephalocele and nasolacrimal duct tumours

b) Mirror or cold spatula misting test to detect condensation and attempted passage of a nasogastric tube.

c) CT paranasal sinuses (includes post nasal space)

d) Persistence of bucconasal membrane or abnormal migration of neural crest cells into nasal vault

e) CHARGE syndrome

   i. **C**oloboma
   ii. **H**eart defects
   iii. **A**tresia of choanae
   iv. **R**etardation of growth and development
   v. **G**enito-renal anomalies
   vi. **E**ar anomalies (external, middle and inner ear deformities)

f) Transnasal and transpalatal approaches; the former requires a 120 degrees Hopkins rigid scope via the oral cavity in order to look at the nasopharyngeal bony/membranous obstruction

1.2 Post-tonsillectomy bleeding in a child

As the surgical SHO you are called to attend an 8-year old child that has had intermittent bleeding following an adenotonsillectomy 12 hours ago for recurrent tonsillitis and persistent glue ear.

Questions

a) According to paediatric life support principles, what would the initial management of this child involve?

b) What blood investigations are appropriate?

c) How are tonsillectomy bleeds classified?

d) If the patient is still bleeding after resuscitation, what are the options? List 4

e) Which new technique has reduced the incidence of post-adenoidectomy bleed to less than 0.5 percent?

Answers

a) Check **A**irways, **B**reathing, **C**irculation and **R**esuscitate.

b) Full blood count, renal profile, Group + Save / Crossmatch, Clotting screen

c) Primary – within 24h, and secondary >24h

d) Attempted control at the bedside using topical haemostatic agents and/or adrenaline (for very mild bleeds); hydrogen peroxide gargle, transfer to theatres for surgical control of bleeding diathermy/cautery, sutures), pack the nasopharynx or oropharynx if necessary for 24 hours in picu.

e) Suction diathermy adenoidectomy

1.3 Syndromes with ENT complications

You are the ENT Doctor reviewing this child in one of your outpatient clinics.

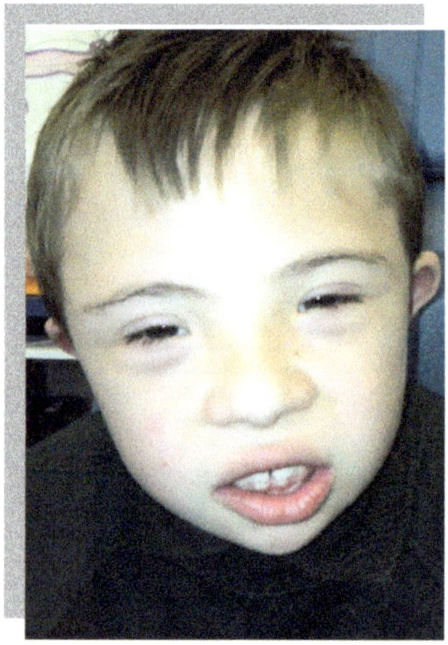

Questions

a) Which syndrome is present in this child shown in the photograph?

b) What is the genetic basis for this condition?

c) List 5 typical physiognomic findings

d) List 8 potential ENT complications that this child may develop

e) Give a non-anatomical reason why this child may have an increased incidence of URTI's

Answers

a) Down syndrome

b) Trisomy 21 due to failure of meiosis, Robertsonian translocation or mosaicism

c) Short neck, up-slanting palpebral fissures, epicanthic folds, hypertelorism, mid-face hypoplasia, single palmar crease, wide nasal gap, small nose, macroglossia, small pinnae

d)

i. Ears: middle ear infections due to ear canal stenosis, otitis media, hearing loss

ii. Nose: Nasal congestion, sinusitis (due to hypoplasic sinuses).

iii. Throat: Obstructive sleep apnoea, Drooling.

iv. Neck: Atlanto-axial instability, stridor and recurrent croup due to subglottic stenosis

e) Association with varying degrees of primary immune dysfunction (reduced/immature T and B cell functions)

1.4 A child with a choking episode

You are called to Emergency Room to see a child who has had an episode of choking. He was playing in the next room when his mother heard him choking and coughing. He is now drooling and has a mild tachypnoea and tachycardia.

Questions

a) List 2 differentials

b) What is your initial management? List 5 steps.

c) What does the following X- ray demonstrate?

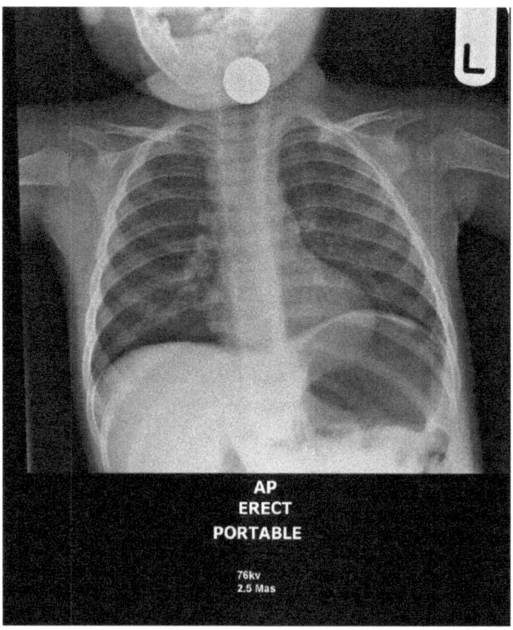

d) What is the most likely anatomical location of this foreign body?

e) What further imaging may be useful?

f) List 5 complications associated with this diagnosis

Answers

a) Swallowed (or less likely inhaled) foreign body

b) **A**irway, **B**reathing, **C**irculation in line with APLS protocol; call for appropriate senior support (paediatric, anaesthetic and ENT); arrange for appropriate imaging

c) Radiodense, circular foreign body in the upper aerodigestive tract. This most likely represents a coin which is the commonest oesophageal foreign body in children.

d) Cricopharyngeus

e) Lateral plain film as well as an abdominal plain film if appropriate (if radiodense object with suspicion of it having gone further down the gastrointestinal tract)

f) Oesophageal perforation, mediastinitis, pneumomediastinum, pneumothorax, aspiration

1.5 A child with stridor

You see a 3-year-old child in A+E who has a 48h history of noisy breathing, pyrexia, agitation and generally being unwell. There is no history of cough. On general inspection she looks very ill and is leaning forward and drooling excessively.

Questions

a) What is the most likely diagnosis?

b) What is your differential?

c) Briefly describe how would you manage this child acutely? Mention at least 5 important points

d) What investigations are necessary?

e) What is the aetiology of this condition and why is it seen less frequently?

Answers

a) Acute epiglottitis

b) Croup, deep neck space infection, severe tonsillitis, impacted foreign body

c) (i) Avoid upsetting the child. (ii) call for immediate Consultant Paediatric anaesthetist and Consultant ENT Surgeon. (iii) Allow the parent to hold nebulised adrenaline in front of the patient. (iv) Arrange calm transfer to theatre where emergency intubation can be performed if necessary. (v) Confirm diagnosis.

d) No investigations are necessary acutely – this may serve to upset the child and result in aspiration of pooled saliva.

e) Classically caused by *Haemophilus Influenza B* – now

rare in UK due to HIB vaccination. Other pathogens include Streptococcus *pneumonia* and beta-haemolytic *Streptococcus, Staphylococcus aureus* and *Haemophilus parainfluenzae*.

1.6 Postoperative note for microlaryngoscopy and bronchoscopy (MLB)

Write a post-operative note for a patient who has undergone a microlaryngoscopy and bronchoscopy (MLB) for recurrent croup. Normal findings are noted

Answer

Date:	25/05/14	Consultant:	Mr J Jones
Patient Details:	James Smith	Surgeon:	Mr EN Throat
Date of Birth:	15/04/2010	Anaesthetist:	Dr I Pain
Hospital No:	x1234567		

Operation:	Microlaryngoscopy and Bronchoscopy
Indication:	Recurrent croup
Findings:	Supraglottis: normal
	Glottis: normal; no laryngeal cleft; normal vocal cord movement (passive and active)
	Subglottis: normal – no evidence of stenosis (normal size as accepted age appropriate ETT)
	Trachea/Bronchi: Normal – no evidence of tracheomalacia; no foreign body seen
Procedure:	General anaesthetic – spontaneous ventilation
	Straight (or curved) laryngoscope used
	4mm 0 degree Hopkins rod used for assessment of airway
Post-op:	Can eat and drink

Observe overnight

If any breathing concerns, inform ENT on-call immediately

Home tomorrow

OPA in 6-8 weeks

1.7 A child with a swelling behind the ear

A 2-year-old child is referred from the emergency room with a swelling behind the right ear

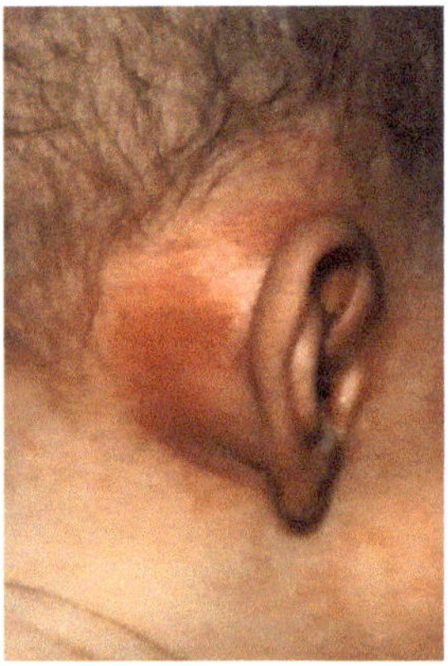

Questions

a) List 5 symptoms that may be present in this child?

b) List 5 signs that may be present in this child?

c) List three differentials of a child with a post-auricular swelling

d) What is the single most important investigation required?

e) List 3 treatment options for this child

This CT scan is performed after 48hours of symptomatic therapy

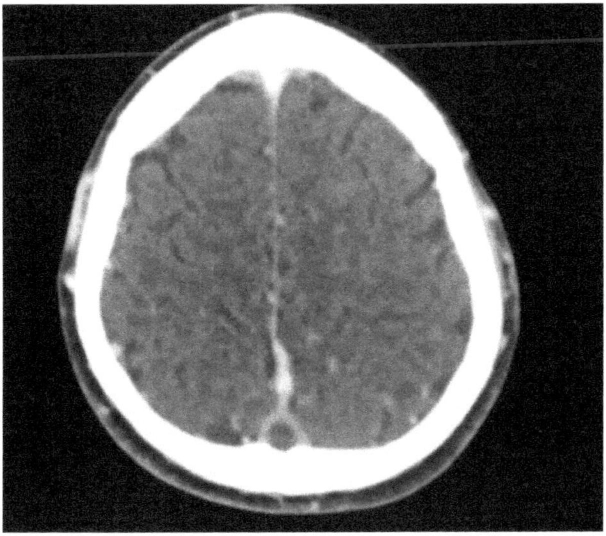

f) What is the main abnormality shown in this scan?

g) What are the other complications of this condition?

Answers

a) Otalgia or ear pulling, otorrhoea, fever, excessive crying, tenderness around mastoid, meningitic symptoms such as stiff neck and headache.

b) Pinna proptosis, fluctuant post-auricular swelling, dull or bulging TM, posterior canal wall sag, lymphadenitis, swelling in occipital area or over sternocleidomastoid, facial nerve palsy.

c) Acute mastoiditis (with possible subperiosteal abscess), post auricular lymphadenopathy, cellulitis, trauma (pinna or mastoid)

d) Contrast CT of temporal bones

e) Initially will require broad spectrum IV antibiotics for 24h. If no improvement or significant systemic illness (+/- neurology) to consider surgical options that include cortical mastoidectomy +/- grommet insertion

f) Axial CT showing 'delta' sign – enhancement of the wall of the sagittal sinus, suggesting cerebral sinus thrombosis

g) Extratemporal, intratemporal (both extracranial) and intracranial

1.8 A child with eye swelling

This 7 year-old presents with a 48hr history of eye swelling

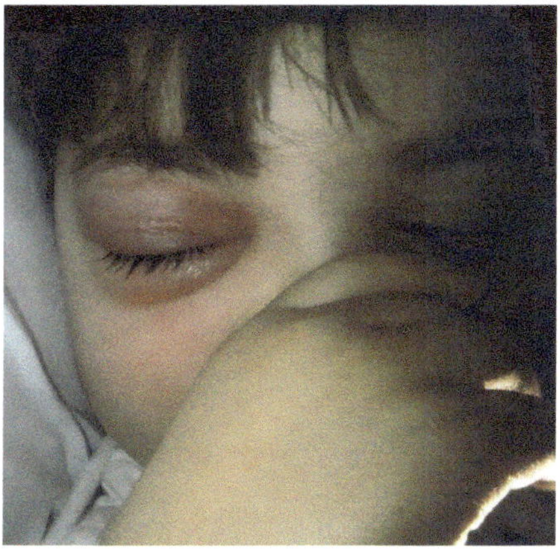

Questions

a) Give 3 differential diagnoses

b) What findings might there be on examination? list 10

c) List three indications for carrying out a CT scan

d) What are the pathophysiological mechanisms leading to this clinical picture? List 3

e) What does the presence of bilateral eye signs indicate?

Answers

a) Periorbital cellulitis, trauma and insect bite

b) General: pyrexia, unwell, malaise

Eyes: proptosis, diplopia, chemosis or pain on eye movement, loss of colour vision

Nose: oedematous nasal mucosa +/- nasal discharge.

Neurology: meningitic symptoms and focal neurology in severe cases

Note that by thinking of the different systems (ie classifying), it is easy to come up with a list of 10 findings

c) Suspicion of post-septal disease; no response to IV antibiotics after 24h; visual acuity cannot be assessed

d) Direct extension (especially if thin walled lamina papyracea), thrombophlebitis (valveless veins), congenital dehiscence, trauma and via lymphatics

e) Cavernous sinus thrombosis

1.9 A painful ear in an upset child

An 18month old child presents to clinic with 12hour history of ear tugging and fever. Upon looking in the ear you see the following:

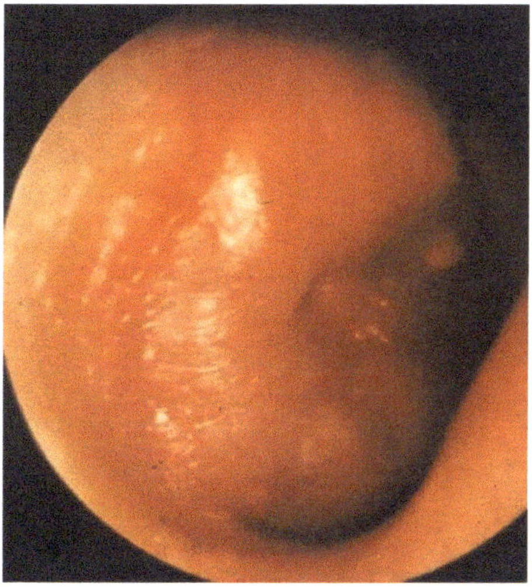

Questions

a) Describe what you see.

b) Which ear is this?

c) What is the likely diagnosis?

d) What are the relative indications for treating this condition with antibiotics from the onset? List 3

e) What is the primary pathophysiological abnormality?

f) What audiometric findings would you expect in this ear?

Answers

a) Bulging and erythematous tympanic membrane

b) Right ear

c) Acute otitis media

d) (i) Children with systemic pathologies such as immunodeficiency, (ii) Under 2 year old, presence of marked systemic upset (i.e. high pyrexia, vomiting), (iii) previous cochlear implantation.

e) Eustachian tube dysfunction results in negative middle ear pressure leading to transudative fluid collection in the middle ear and subsequent infection

f) Tympanogram: Type B (flat trace)

   Audiogram: Conductive hearing loss (maximum 60dB)

1.10 A child with a hoarse voice

Flexible nasendoscopy is performed on a 10 year old

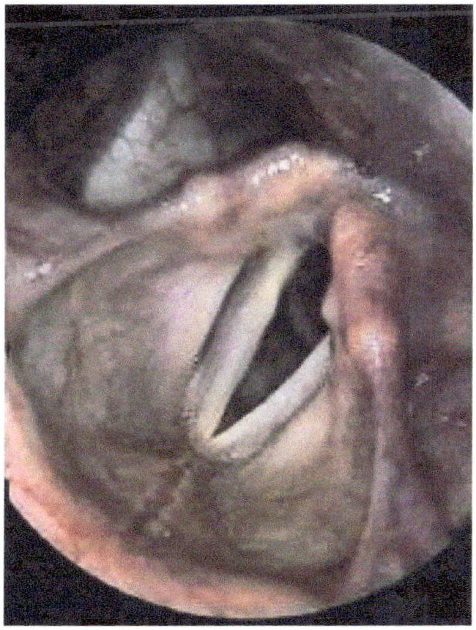

Questions

a. What is the diagnosis?

b. List 3 common causes for this pathology in a child

c. Give 2 symptoms this child may have?

d. How would you manage this problem in a child. List 3 options

e. List 3 causes for bilateral pathology.

Answers

a. Left vocal cord palsy

b. Congenital, intubation, iatrogenic , i.e. from birth or surgical trauma (e.g.PDA ligation or aortic arch anomaly repair or tracheoesophageal fistula repair)

c. Hoarse-breathy dysphonia, aspiration/feeding difficulties (including dysphagia). Other symptoms may include stridor and vocal fatigue

d. If asymptomatic, no active management may be needed. For children with voice problems speech and language therapy is required. For children with feeding difficulties NG tube insertion or even a PEG tube maybe required. If recurrent aspiration is the problem, for neonates or young children a tracheostomy has to be considered. Note that surgery to the vocal cords is rarely done in the paediatric group unless there is a separate pathological process going on.

e. Neurologic (Arnold-Chiari malformation and meningomyelocele), iatrogenic (birth trauma, increased risk with forceps or complicated delivery), idiopathic

1.11 A child with hearing problems

This 4-year old girl is seen in clinic with her parents who have concerns with her hearing and language development. She fails to respond to commands consistently, sits very close to the TV and is not as advanced as her older siblings when they were at the same stage. On otoscopy the following is seen:

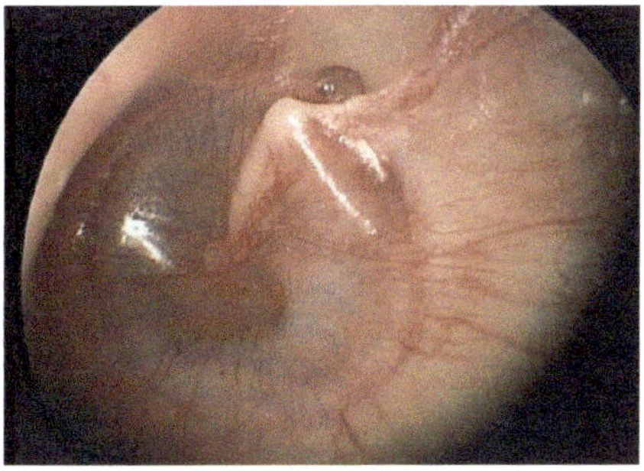

Questions

a) What is the diagnosis?

b) List 10 important questions that should be covered in the history?

c) List two appropriate investigations

d) What three features in the photograph support the diagnosis?

e) What non-surgical options are there to manage this condition?

f) What are the 2 recommended surgical procedures to treat this condition?

g) Name 3 conditions which may be associated with refractory disease.

Answers

a) Otitis media with effusion

b) Length of history (>3months), speech delay, balance disturbance, pain, history of AOM, nasal problems/blockage, snoring/OSA, sore throats, chest infections, birth history, other infections / immune deficits

c) PTA or age appropriate hearing assessment, tympanogram

d) Retracted tympanic membrane, dull appearance and neo-annulus

e) Watch and wait 3 months, autoinflation, hearing aids, steroid therapy

f) Ventilation tube insertion and adenoidectomy

g) (i) Submucous cleft, (ii) impaired mucociliary clearances (e.g. primary ciliary dyskinesia); (iii) autoimmune screen (e.g. Wegener's)

1.12 Skin prick allergy testing

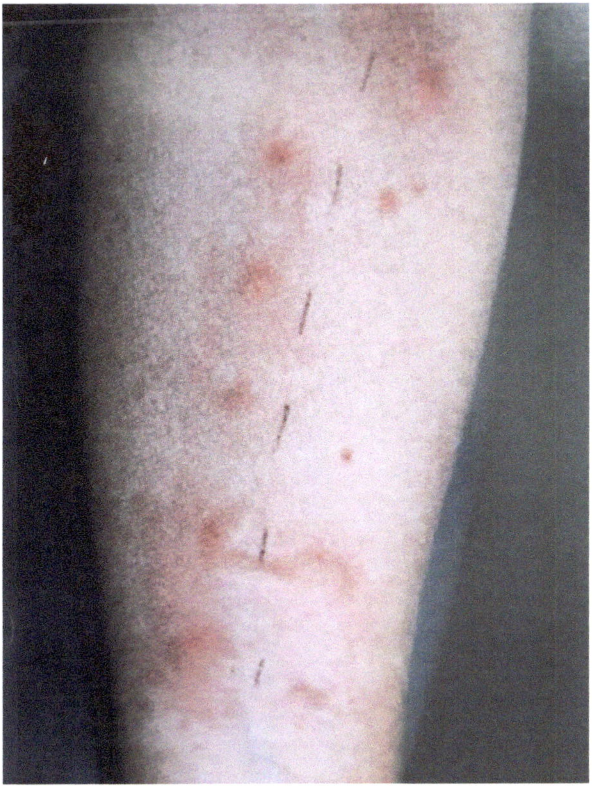

Questions

a) What test is being done here?

b) When is the test positive?

c) What are 3 contraindications

d) List 6 common aero-allergens.

e) What is the signigicance of a positive wheal with control?

f) What is the full name of the alternative test using a blood sample and what does the test measure?

Answers

a) Skin prick allergy test

b) Wheal present after 15 minutes. Has to be compared to negative control – 2mm children, 3mm adults

c) High or known risk of anaphylaxis, skin disorders (severe eczema, dermatographia), unco-operative patient (e.g. child or infants), antihistamines 48-72hrs prior to testing (increased risk of false negatives)

d) House dust, house dust mites (faeces), animal dander, tree (birch, alder, cedar), grass, weeds, fungi and spores

e) Test is void because the patient is reacting to the vehicle used to carry the allergen

f) RAST – radioallergosorbent test; measures IgE level

1.13 A snoring child

A child who snores loudly at night is referred to clinic. On inspection of the oral cavity the following is seen:

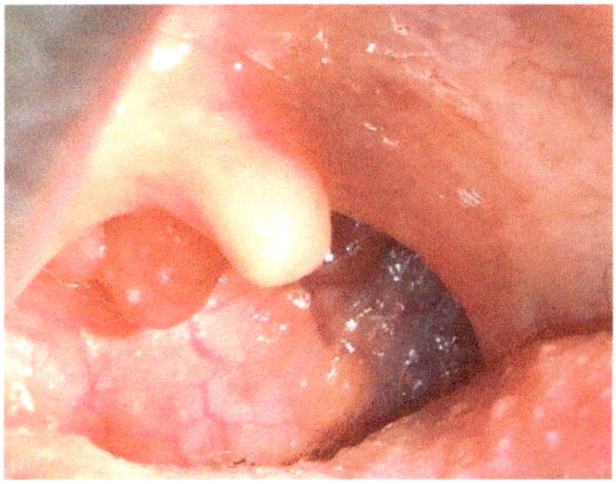

Questions

a) Describe the finding

b) What symptoms might this child be experiencing? List 5

c) What condition may exacerbate or perpetuate these symptoms?

d) What other condition is this child very likely to have?

e) What operation might the child benefit from?

f) What postoperative instructions would you give? List 4.

Answers

a) Large adenoid protruding from the nasopharynx into the oropharynx

(note that adenoid pad is singular not plural)

b) Snoring, daytime somnolence, recurrent ear infections, purulent rhinorrhea, halitosis/malodorous breath, hyponasal speech, post nasal drip

c) In children, gastro-oesophageal reflux can lead to chronic adenoiditis

d) Otitis media with effusion

e) Adenoidectomy (tonsils already removed)

f) Regular observations post-operatively; overnight stay only if very small, afternoon list, significant OSA that would require post-operative oxygen saturation measurements; regular analgesia and antibiotics for a week; follow-up arrangements

1.14 A child with nasal regurgitation

Questions

a) List 5 symptoms associated with velopharyngeal insufficiency

b) List 3 common causes

c) List 3 other members of the multidisciplinary team that may be involved in the care of such patients

d) What are the treatment options

e) List 4 surgical complications

Answers

a) Hypernasal speech, nasal regurgitation, impaired speech intelligibility, increased nasal resonance and decreased speech volume

b) Syndrome associated (e.g. Di-George syndrome - 22q11 is the classic one), submucous cleft palate, iatrogenic (after adenoidectomy or cleft palate repair)

c) Cleft/plastic surgeon, speech and language therapist, psychologist

d) Speech and language therapy, surgery (e.g. Furlow palatoplasty, superior-based pharyngeal flap, sphincter pharyngoplasty, prosthetic obturation)

e) Obstructive sleep apnoea, aspiration/pneumonia, haemorrhage (be aware of medialised carotids in 22q11 patients), nasopharyngeal stenosis, neck stiffness, hyponasality

1.15 Sore throat

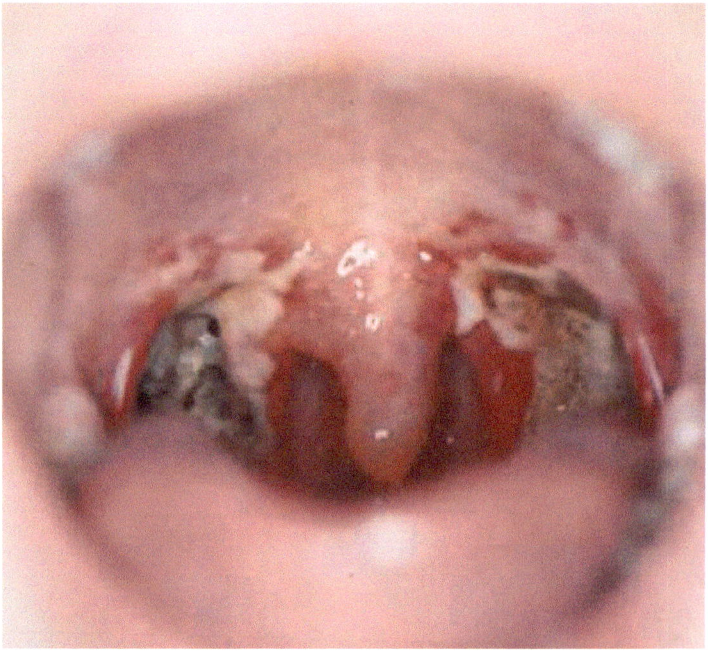

Questions

a) What procedure has been performed here?

b) List 4 techniques that may be used when performing this procedure

c) List 8 complications of this procedure

d) What would you have to consider when performing this case on a Down's syndrome patient

e) Name 6 surgical instruments you would require for this procedure

Answers

a) Tonsillectomy

b) Cold steel, diathermy (bipolar or monopolar), coblation, laser

c) Pain (often associated with dehydration), nausea and vomiting (usually anaesthetic complication), bleeding, infection, damage to teeth/lips, change in quality of voice (if older child/adolescent), post-operative airway compromise, no improvement of symptoms

d) Care with neck due to risk of atlanto-axial subluxation. Keep patient in neutral position.

e) Boyle-Davis gag, Draffin rods, Dennis-Browne forceps, Gwynne-Evans tonsil dissector, Mollison's pillar retractor, Curved Negus clamp, Negus knot pusher

1.16 Laryngeal lesions

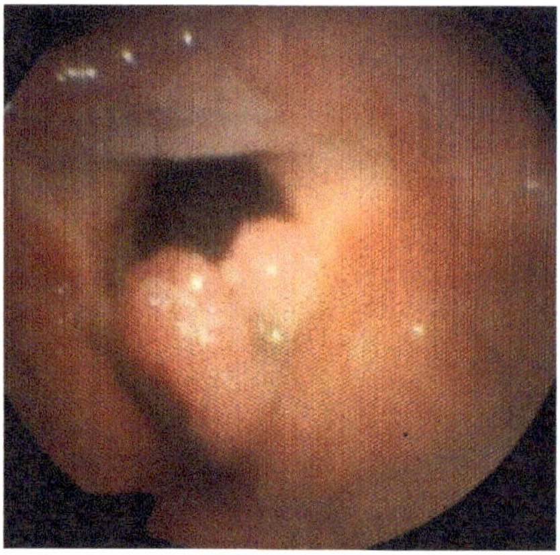

Questions

a) List 3 causes of chronic hoarseness in the paediatric population?

b) How would you assess a child in clinic with chronic hoarseness? List 5 things

c) What would be your management options for this condition? List 5

d) What is the principle of surgical management and why?

e) List 3 factors that can contribute to malignant transformation.

Answers

a) Vocal cord nodules (commonest); recurrent respiratory papillomatosis (second commonest); vocal fold paralysis; post-surgical (laryngotracheal reconstruction)

b) History: include principle symptoms and chronicity (e.g.

voice/cry, time of onset) neonatal history (including intubation), lower respiratory and upper respiratory symptoms, feeding, other medical problems/procedures, maternal/paternal history of genital condylomata.

Examination: include intra-oral examination as well as endoscopy (2.4-4mm depending on age of child) assessing nose and upper aerodigestive tract

c) Conservative (wait and watch with regular follow ups)

Medical: (adjuvant chemical therapy and so rarely used as sole treatment: (e.g. indol–3 carbinol, alpha interferon, cidofovir; ribavirin, acyclovir, cimetidine.

Surgical: microdebridement (gold standard), cold steel, laser (CO_2, KTP, Nd:Yag, flash pump dye laser)

d) Aim of treatment is to improve airway and voice while decreasing spread and preserving normal structures Aggressive treatment should be avoided because of risk of glottic or subglottic stenosis and laryngeal webbing

e) History of radiation, smoking, HPV types 16/18

1.17 A stridulous infant

This is the larynx of a baby with stridor.

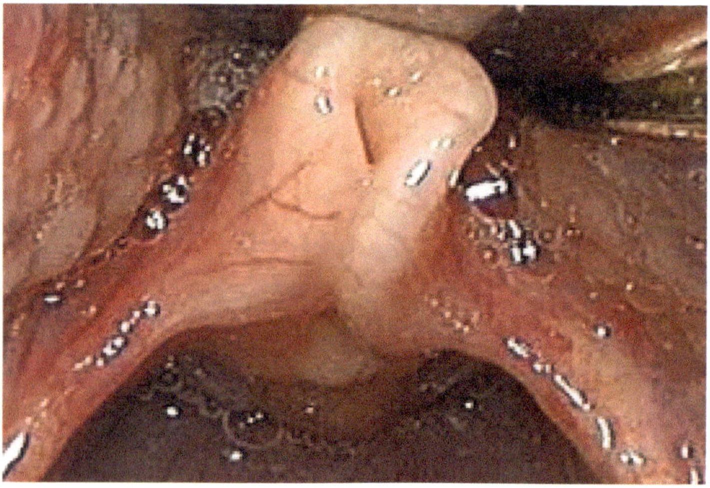

Questions

a) What is the most likely diagnosis?

b) What might exacerbate or improve the stridor?

c) List 5 other symptoms/signs the child might present with?

d) List 3 common surgical findings that explain the stridor

e) What surgical procedure is the mainstay of treatment in severe cases?

Answers

a) Laryngomalacia because of curled over-riding epiglottis (omega epiglottis)

b) Worse on exertion (feeding, crying) or supine position, Better with prone position

c) Feeding difficulties poor weight gain, failure to thrive, sternocostal recession, tracheal tug

d) Short aryepiglottic folds with inwards inspiratory collapse; excessive mucosa over arytenoid and cuneiform-corniculate complex; long, tubular epiglottis with posterior placement

e) Supraglottoplasty (aka aryepiglottoplasty)

1.18 Child with noisy breathing and recurrent URTI

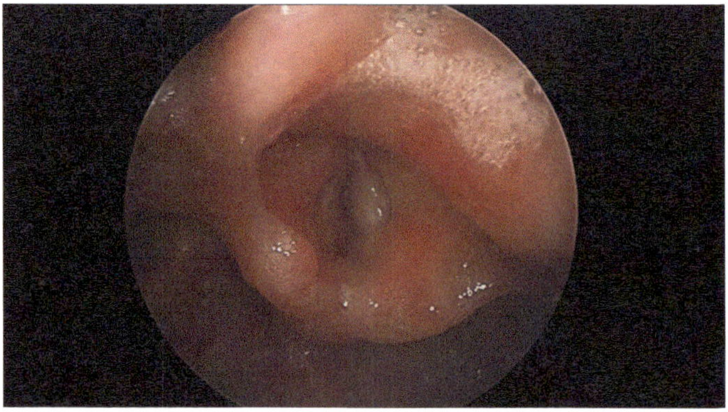

Questions

a) What is the most likely diagnosis?

b) List 3 presenting symptoms

c) How is this condition graded?

d) How is this condition diagnosed?

e) How is this condition treated? List 4 options

Answers

a) Subglottic stenosis (Endoscopic photograph of a severe pin point subglottic stenosis in a child)

b) Biphasic stridor; croup/recurrent URTIs; failure to thrive, acute airway obstruction (in extremis)

c) Cotton-Meyer grading scale (I: <50% obstruction; II: 51-70% obstruction; III 71-99% obstruction; IV: no detectable lumen)

d) Microlaryngoscopy and bronchoscopy

e) Conservative (if less severe stenosis and asymptomatic patient); dilatation with a balloon (see post op picture below); medical: anti-reflux medication (often as an adjunct treatment); surgical: cricoid split; laryngotracheal resection; cricotrachea resection; tracheotomy

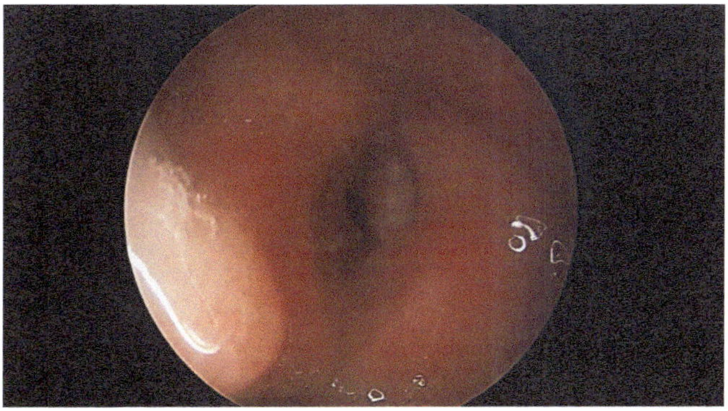

1.19 Child presenting with aspiration pneumonia

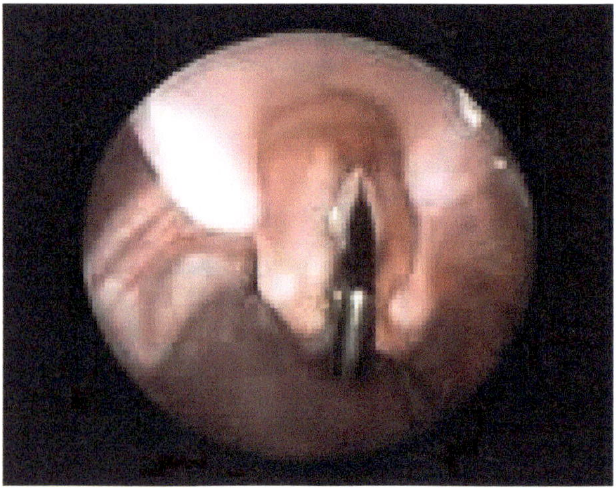

Questions

a) What is the diagnosis?

b) List 4 symptoms this patient may present with

c) What investigations are relevant in this case? List 3

d) List 3 treatment options

Answers

a) Laryngeal cleft

b) Aspiration with feeding; respiratory difficulties; gastro-oesophageal reflux; occasional stridor; weak voice; increased tracheal secretions

c) (i) MLB – diagnostic; (ii) CXR – for any respiratory complications; (iii) Water soluble contrast to look for a trachea-oesophageal fistula

d) (i) Conservative – no treatment; (ii) medical – aggressive reflux treatment; optimise nutritional and pulmonary status;(iii) Surgical – cleft repair; tracheostomy

1.20 A bleeding ear

A 5-year old boy is brought to the Emergency Department (ED) by his parents with a bleeding, bruised and swollen right ear. His Mother stated to the triage nurse that he fell onto that side 5 days ago and it has only now started bleeding and become swollen. When the ED registrar assessed the child, his Father stated that he had been hit in the ear at school yesterday. When you see the child, Mum is not sure of how the injury occurred, or when it had occurred. On examination, you notice a fresh bruise over his right pinna and mastoid area and an older bruise around his left eye. There is dried blood at his right external meatus. The father states that the eye bruise occurred at school. The child does not talk to you.

Questions

a) Describe the otoscopic finding

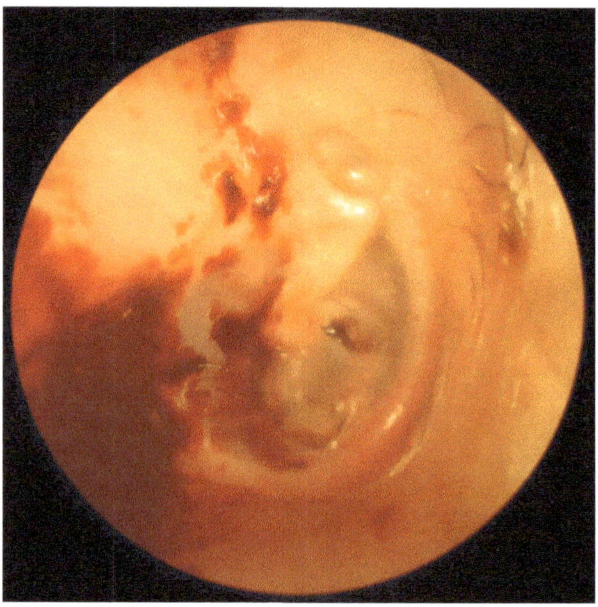

b) List 6 differential diagnoses

c) What is the main concern in the history

d) How would you manage this patient?

Answers

a) Right tympanic membrane with an anterior perforation. The pars tensa appears also retracted. There is a haematoma of the posterior wall of the ear canal and blood crusts in the canal

b) Non-accidental injury (NAI); blunt ear trauma; pinna haematoma; underlying coagulopathy; epilepsy, balance disorder leading to falls; otitis media with perforation

c) The concern is of a NAI – inconsistencies in the story and the 'frozen watchfulness' in a post-lingual child. Over-familiarity is also a concerning sign in a child and may signal neglect.

d) If NAI concern:

Inform the Responsible Officer of the Child Protection Team at the hospital; this is usually a Paediatric doctor

Admit the child to hospital to allow time to contact the local child protection services

Exclude all other possible diagnoses

It is important not to overlook clinical needs: in this case consider topical antibiotics and aural toilet to remove crusts.

1.21 A drooling child

You are asked to see a 4-year-old child. His mother is concerned about his face and clothes being regularly soiled by saliva

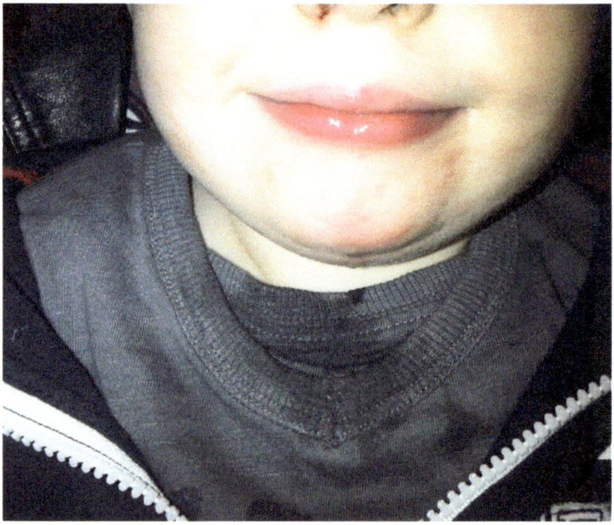

Questions

a) What is this condition?

b) Above what age is it considered abnormal?

c) List 5 causes for this problem

d) How would you assess this chid? List 4 things

e) How could you very broadly classify this condition?

f) List 10 management options

Answers

a) Drooling

b) 5 years of age

c) Neurological (cerebral palsy, neurological immaturity with poor oromotor control, developmental delay)

   Hypersecretion (inflammatory, parasympathomimetic medications, GORD)

   Psychogenic

   Anatomical (macroglossia, orthodontic problems, nasal obstruction)

d) History: number of bibs/clothing changes per day, developmental milestones, dental problems, recurrent pneumonia, impact on family and quality of life

   Examination: Exclude acute causes (e.g. foreign bodies, infections), adenotonsillar assessment; syndromic features

e) Acute drooling: (e.g. foreign body, infections such as epiglottitis, tonsillitis, gingivitis)

   Chronic drooling (e.g. cerebral palsy, syndromic children, children on anti-convulsants)

f) Conservative: reassurance, speech and language therapy; orthodontist

   Medical: botulinum toxin injection, anticholinergic medications, radiation therapy

   Surgical: submandibular gland excision, parotid duct ligation, submandibular duct/parotid duct rerouting, adenotonsillectomy, Jacobson's nerve neurectomy

1.22 An unwell child post-tonsillectomy

You are asked to see a 3-year old boy who underwent adenotonsillectomy for OSA 3 days previously. He is pale and lethargic but afebrile with a HR of 165bpm, respiratory rate 40min and capillary refill time of 5 seconds, BP is 60/40mmHg. This patient is shocked.

Questions

a) What is the clinical definition of shock?

b) What kind of shock is this?

c) What is the most concerning aspect of this child's vital signs?

d) How would you manage this child? List 5 things

e) If this child was pyrexial, how would your management be altered?

f) If vascular access is not achievable, how else might fluid be administered to this patient?

Answers

a) Shock refers to systemic organ dysfunction resulting from hypo-perfusion and/or hypo-oxygenation

b) In this case it is from hypovolaemia due to blood loss

c) Low BP is a pre-terminal sign of decompensation and circulatory collapse may quickly follow

d) **A** – clear clots and administer high flow oxygen,

   B – assess effort, efficacy and effect of breathing,

   C – reassess signs and urine output and obtain 2 wide bore IV access lines whilst obtaining blood for crossmatch, FBC, coagulopathy screen. Administer a 20ml/kg non-dextrose containing fluid bolus and check for response. If bleeding continues and once 40ml/kg had been administered, colloid/blood products may be given next. Once stabilised the child should be taken to theatre to formally control the bleed

e) Pyrexia suggests an infective component i.e. septic shock. Administration of a third generation cephalosporin would be appropriate e.g. ceftriaxone.

f) Intraosseous infusion

1.23 Lip deformity

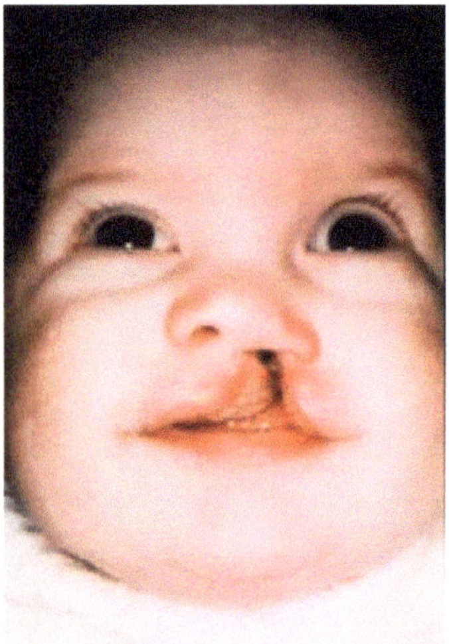

Questions

a) What does the picture show?

b) What would your examination focus on?

c) What classification system exists for this condition

d) Name 4 healthcare professionals that will be involved in the care of this child

e) What is a submucosal cleft?

f) How might this be relevant to an ENT surgeon?

Answers

a) Unilateral cleft lip

b) Oral examination to determine extent and palatal

integrity. Should also examine for other craniofacial, nasal and otological defects.

c) Veau classification of palatal cleft:

   i. Class 1 – isolated soft palate

   ii. Class 2 – isolated hard palate

   iii. Class 3 - unilateral cleft lip and palate

   iv. Class 4 – bilateral cleft lip and palate

d) Speech and language therapist, orthodontist, facial plastics and cleft surgeon

e) Failure of midline fusion of the soft palate musculature. Typically associated with a bifid uvula and midline notching of the free border of the hard palate. May result in weakness of the Eustachian tube dilators, increasing the risk of recurrent OME.

f) An adenoidectomy in such patients may lead to velopalatal insufficiency

CHAPTER 2

Rhinology

2.1 A chef with a serious problem

A 35-year old chef presents to your clinic with a change in his ability to smell or taste foods.

Questions

a) List 5 things you would ask in the history

b) What is the single most important examination would you would perform in clinic?

c) List two appropriate investigations

d) List 3 things that you would include in your differential

e) What modality is the following image and what does it show?

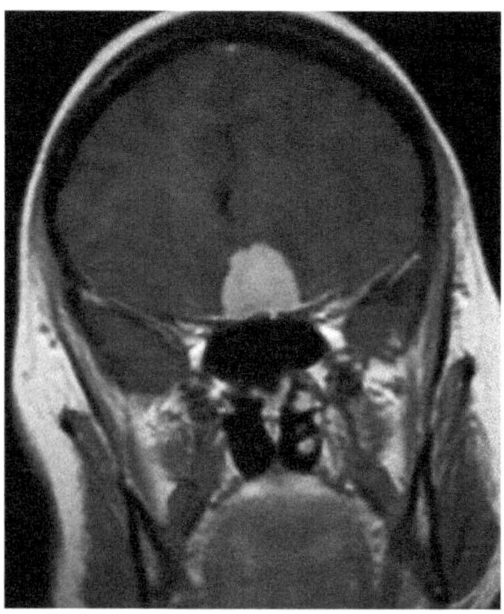

f) What important home safety steps need to be taken?

Name 3.

Answers

a) Other rhinitic symptoms (epistaxis, nasal obstruction, nasal discharge, facial pains, allergy/itching), recent URTI, head injury, infertility (Kallman's syndrome)

b) Rigid nasendoscopy with a Hopkins endoscope to assess anatomy of nose, including its roof (cribiform plate between the septum and middle turbinate) to exclude any mucosal disease or masses (Anosmia is classified in the same way as hearing loss: conductive or sensorineural)

c) UPSIT (University of Pennsylvania Smell identification test, also known as scratch and sniff test), MRI brain

d) Anything that disrupts the pathway between olfactory cells and the brain (i.e., nasal blockage, viral infection, basal skull fracture, tumour)

e) T1 Contrast-enhanced MRI coronal section, showing an enhancing broad-based lesion in the olfactory region, consistent with a diagnosis of meningioma

f) Check food sell by dates, fit smoke alarms, change gas cooker to electric

2.2 Recurrent epistaxis

You are referred a Egyptian teenager boy by a GP who has a history of recurrent epistaxis and unilateral nasal obstruction.

Questions

a) Describe the scan below

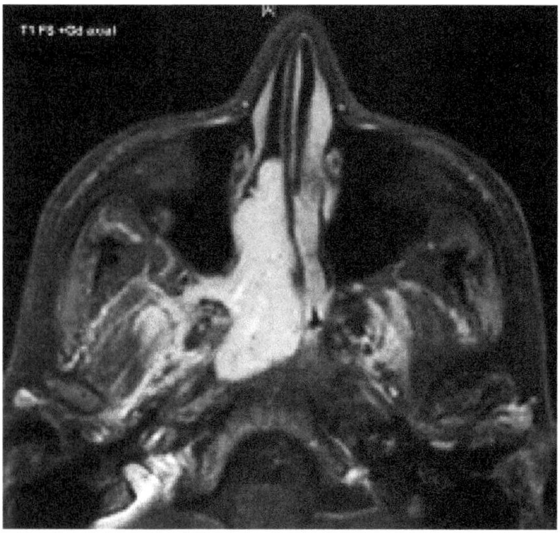

b) What is the most likely diagnosis?

c) List 4 complications associated with this condition

d) What is the main blood supply to this lesion?

e) List 3 treatment options

f) What procedure may be helpful before surgery?

Answers

a) MRI T1 weighted image through the nasal cavity showing a high signal lesion in the right nasal cavity and nasopharynx with extension into the vidian canal.

b) Juvenile nasal angiofibroma (JNA)

c) Significant bleeding; extension into sinuses (with associated sinusitis), orbit (blindness, diplopia, proptosis); intracranial and skull base extension

d) Internal maxillary artery

e) Endoscopic surgery, open surgical approaches (e.g. midface degloving), radiation and chemotherapy, hormonal therapy (e.g. oestrogen)

f) Embolisation of the feeding vessel

2.3 Nasal trauma

This patient presents to your clinic having sustained an injury to her nose 2 days previously when she fell over under the influence of alcohol.

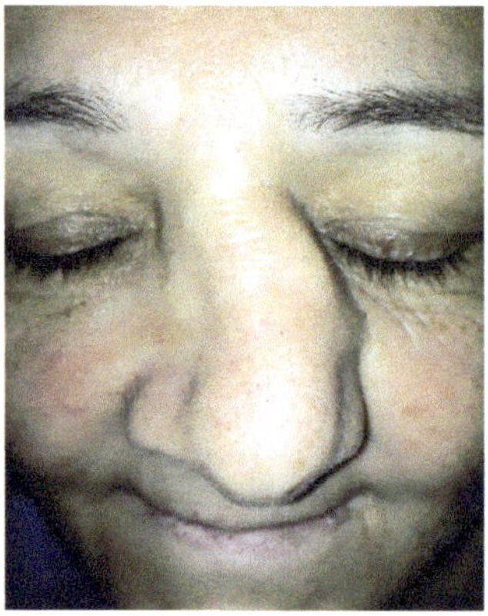

Questions

a) Describe the abnormalities

b) How is this condition classified?

c) What important points are there to take in the history? List 5

d) When is the best time to review these patients?

e) What important complication is it vital to exclude in the examination?

f) What would be the options for surgical management?

g) What does this management not address?

h) What complications would you put on the consent form? List 5

Answers

a) Leftward deviation of the nasal bone, depressed on the right. No overlying laceration

b) Type 1: frontal blow causing depressed or displaced distal portion of nasal bone. Associated vertical septal fracture

   Type 2: Lateral trauma with lateral deviation of nasal bones and associated horizontal or C-shaped septal fracture

   Type 3: Severe trauma with fracture of ethmoids; collapse of septum into face.

c) How trauma was acquired (eg domestic abuse), presence of nasal obstruction, rhinorrhoea, and visual problems (blowout fracture diplopia), head injury symptoms

d) First hour of trauma or 7-10 days after the incident allowing for local oedema to subside

e) Septal haematoma

f) Manipulation under anaesthesia (MUA) – local or general anaesthetic

g) MUA will not resolve a septal deviation (particularly important if the deviation is causing nasal obstruction and significant cosmetic deformity)

h) Infection, bleeding and need for nasal packing, discomfort/pain, need for further surgery (further MUA or septorhinoplasty), imperfect result/nasal deformity

2.4 Skin lesion on the nose

The following patient presents to outpatients with a lesion of 3 month's standing on the lateral aspect of the nose

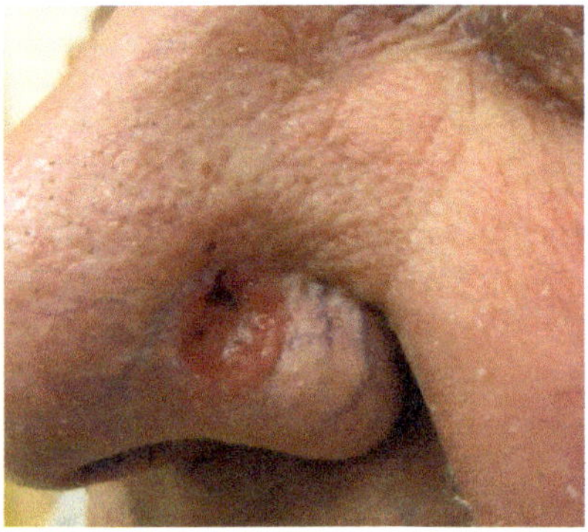

Questions

a) Describe the photograph

b) Name two differential diagnoses other than BCC

c) How is the definitive diagnosis made?

d) Histology confirms BCC - What available reconstructive options are suitable? List 4

e) State 2 non-surgical management options

Answers

a) Photograph showing a well circumscribed lesion with an ulcerated centre on the left alar cartilage

b) SCC, Papilloma

c) Excision biopsy

d) Reconstruction ladder: secondary intention, primary closure, split thickness skin graft, full thickness skin graft, local flap

e) Radiotherapy or cryosurgery

2.5 A nasal lesion

A 20 year-old gentleman presents to your clinic with unilateral nasal obstruction.

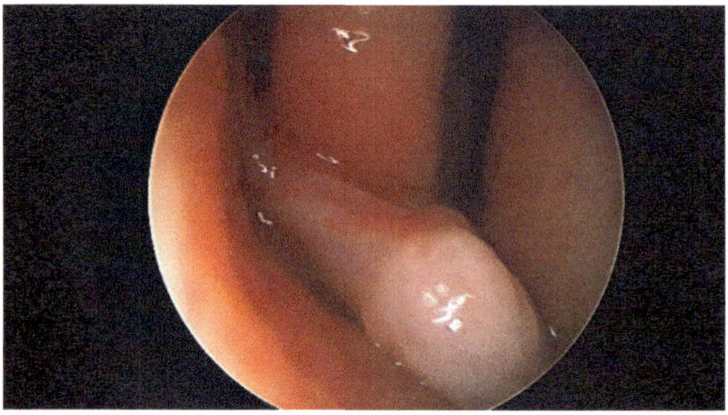

Questions

a. What is the pathology shown in the clinical photograph above?

b. List 10 things you would include your history would include

c. Other than examination of the nose, list 2 other things you would assess

d. What needs to be excluded in this case?

e. List the next 2 essential steps in the management of this patient

f. Should this patient undergo endoscopic sinus surgery, what else would you include in the consent form?

Answers

a. Nasal polyp that most likely represents an antrochoanal

polyp

b. Other rhinitic symptoms (epistaxis, smell, rhinorrhea, facial pain, itchy nose); timing of presenting complaint; past medical history (including allergy/hayfever, asthma); medications (asking specifically about aspirin and allergies to medications); social history (including smoking, pets, social circumstances)

c. Intraoral and oropharyngeal examination; palpation of neck for other masses/nodes

d. Unilateral nasal polyposis in an adult is always suspicious of a malignancy.

e. CT/MRI scan and tissue diagnosis or formal endoscopic sinus surgery

f. Consent for Caldwell-Luc incision as endoscopic access to disease in the anterior maxillary sinus may be difficult.

2.6 A nosebleed

A 60 year old is referred with intermittent nosebleeds that settle with first-aid measures. They are usually left sided.

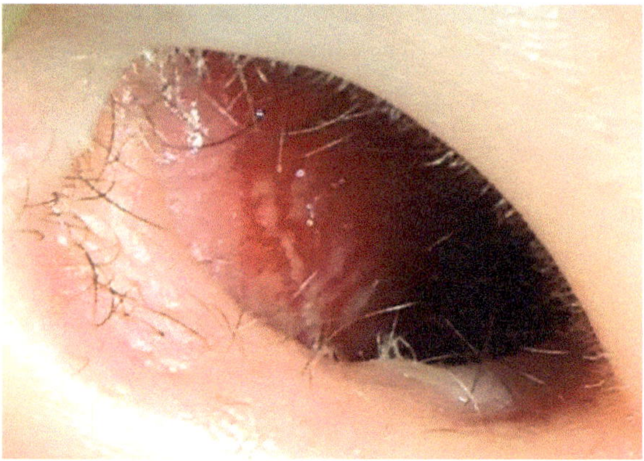

Questions

a) Describe the image shown in the clinical photograph

b) How would you manage an acute episode of this condition? List 3 things

c) If there is no response to this, what steps should be taken? List 3

d) What operative options can be used if the epistaxis persists? List 3

e) What is Woodruff's plexus?

f) What steps can you take to reduce the risk of this condition recurring? List 3

Answers

a) Anterior rhinoscopy of left septum demonstrating multiple vessels in Little's area/Kiesselbach's plexus

b) Pressure (pinching the soft part of the nose), ice pack over neck followed by anterior rhinoscopy and haemostasis with silver nitrate sticks or electrocautery

c) If this fails pack nose , obtain IV access and take bloods (inc G+S), resuscitate as needed, oral antibiotics if packs to remain for more than 24h (failure to control bleeding may occur if the patient has deranged clotting eg due to anti-coagulation medications)

d) Sphenopalatine artery ligation, maxillary artery ligation or external carotid artery ligation (extreme cases). Embolization (usually of maxillary artery) is an alternative

e) Common source of posterior bleeds. Confluence of vessels (mainly from the sphenopalatine artery) on lateral wall, posterior to inferior and middle turbinates

f) Review anticoagulants, counsel patient (factors contributing to nose bleeds and primary measures to stop them), optimise blood pressure, prescribe Naseptin

2.7 Septal surgery

Questions

a) List the three components of the septum

b) Name 5 arteries supplying the nasal septum.

c) What is the basic histology of the nasal septum?

d) What incisions may be used when operating on the nasal septum? Describe where you would make them?

e) List one advantage and disadvantage for each of these incisions

f) Which is the importance of keystone area of the nose?

g) List the 4 components of the key stone area.

Answers

a) Membraneous, cartilaginous and bony septum

b) Anterior ethmoidal, posterior ethmoidal, superior labial, greater palatine and posterior septal (one of the terminal branches of the sphenopalatine artery – the other terminal branch is the posteriolateral nasal artery to the lateral nasal wall)

c) Predominantly respiratory epithelium, with a small area of olfactory epithelium extending from cribriform plate onto upper septum. Submucosal layer containing seromucinous glands and goblet cells (mucus production); Bowman's glands are only present with olfactory epithelium. Overall, nasal septum sandwiched on either side by mucoperiosteal and mucoperichondrial flaps.

d) Killian's incision (a mucosal incision 1-1.5cm behind the caudal edge of the septum) and hemitransfixion incision (J-shaped vestibular incision over caudal free edge of cartilage extending from the floor of nasal cavity to the dorsal tip at the caudal end of the septum).

e) Killian's incision helps to get into correct sub-pericondrial plane easily but not indicated for addressing caudal septal defects, such as collumellar dislocation. It is more challenging to get into the right plane with a hemitransfixion incision but gives access to the most caudal end of the septum and anterior nasal spine for re-securing the septum

f) The Keystone area of the nose is very important during nasal surgery to maintain the stability of the nose and to prevent dorsal collapse (saddle nose).

g) It consists of the area formed by the paired nasal bone cephalically, paired upper lateral cartilage, quadrangular cartilage anterior-inferiorly and the perpendicular plate of the ethmoid bone postero-inferiorly.

2.8 Intracranial complications of sinusitis

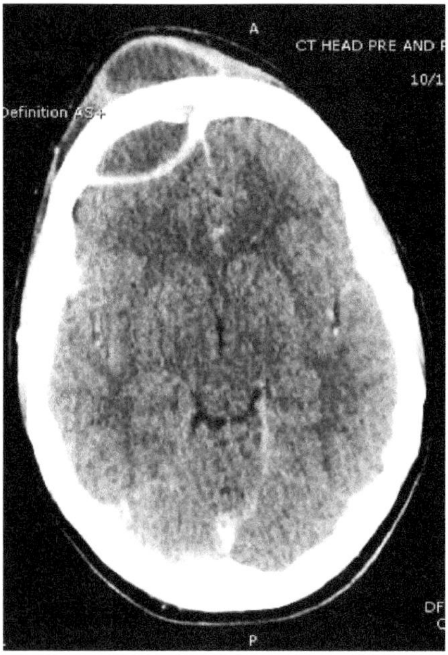

Questions

a) What is the image above and what does it show?

b) What is the eponymous name for this condition?

c) How can a sinusitis infection spread and cause intracranial complications? List 3 routes

d) What types of intracranial complications are you aware of? List 5

e) How may a patient present? List 5 possible symptoms

f) How would you manage such a patient? List 5 basic

steps

g) What are the treatment options? List 3

Answers

a) Axial CT head (soft tissue window) showing a swelling over the frontal bone with corresponding intracerebral ring-enhancing lesion that most likely represent an intracerebral abscess

b) Pott's puffy tumour

c) Direct extension via osteomyelitic bone; via venous channels or general haematogenous spread (rare); via traumatic bone disruption

d) Meningitis; epidural or subdural abscess; intracranial abscess (frontal lobe); cavernous sinus thrombosis associated with sphenoid sinus thrombosis; otitic hydrocephalus via sagittal sinus thrombosis; subdural empyema

e) Symptoms may be mild and non-specific such as headache and fever as well as nausea and vomiting. Nuchal rigidity may indicate meningitis and any drop in GCS/increased confusion could indicate a serious intracranial complication. Ocular symptoms may also be present such as decreased visual acuity, ophthalmoplegia as well as blindness. Focal neurology is rare.

f)

   i. History: Evaluate symptoms and relevant timings; relevant ENT past medical history

ii. Examination: Complete ear, nose (endoscopic), throat and head and neck assessment. Assessment of cranial nerves. Basic neurological exam and eye assessment

iii. Relevant investigations: Basic bloods (FBC, CRP, clotting, U&Es); blood cultures; LP may be needed but after CT scan.

iv. Imaging: CT/MRI

v. In such cases, the ENT surgeon should promptly involve other colleagues. A neurosurgical opinion is needed when abscesses are present. If meningitis is the presenting problem, neurology input is needed. Any opthalmological/orbital pathology will require input from the ophthalmologists

g) **Medical**: high dose intravenous antibiotics, +/- anti-coagulation. **Surgical**: sinus surgery (endoscopic or open). Any intracranial collection to be drained by neurosurgeon

2.9 Bilateral intranasal lesions

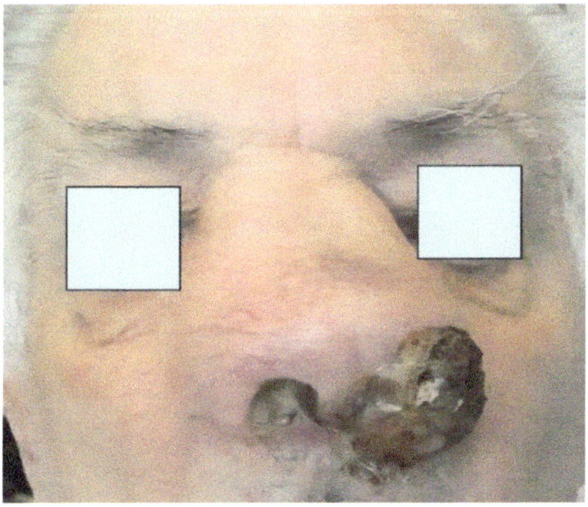

Questions

a) What would be your most likely diagnosis considering the lesion and the shape of the nose?

b) List four likely aetiological factors

c) List 4 differentials if this patient was a 5 year-old

d) In unilateral cases, list 3 important differentials

e) What investigation would you request following your initial assessment?

Answers

a) Nasal (sinonasal) polyposis

b) (i) Allergy (e.g. allergic rhinitis); (ii) Vasomotor (no identified allergen); (iii) Inflammation (i.e. post viral or bacterial illness); (iv) Genetic (including Samter's triad that includes aspirin intolerance, late onset asthma in the presence of nasal polyps)

c) (i) Cystic fibrosis (the most likely) (ii) Kartagener's syndrome (iii) Immunodeficiency (iv) Coeliac disease

d) (i) Neoplastic process (e.g. inverted papilloma, SCC, adenocarcinoma); (ii) Antrochoanal polyp; (iii) Encephalocoele/meningocoele/glioma

e) CT and if considering glioma/encephalocoele/meningocoele an MRI

2.10 Persistent rhinosinusitis

A GP refers you this patient: *Please could you kindly see this 42 year old lady with a history of recurrent episodes of sinusitis, occurring 4 times each winter, requiring antibiotics on each occasion and which is now causing her significant symptoms. A CT scan has been organised.*

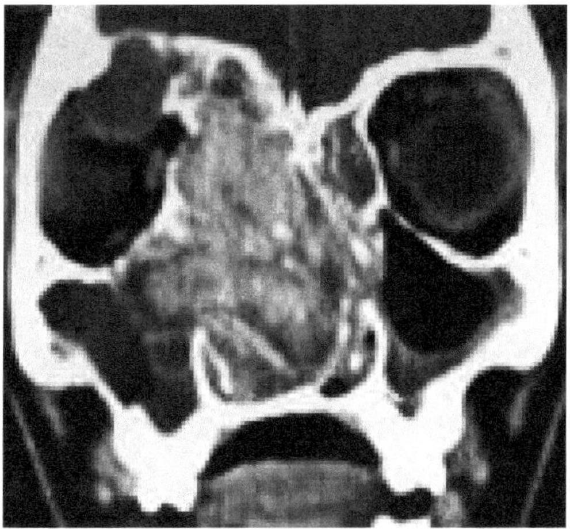

Questions

a) Describe the image

b) List 4 important differentials?

c) How is fungal sinusitis diagnosed?

d) How is it classified?

e) What role is there for antifungal agents?

Answers

a) Coronal CT scan of the nose and paranasal sinuses,

showing unilateral opacification of the right maxillary, ethmoid sinuses. There is a large expansive mass within the right side of the nose leading to extensive bony invasion. There appears to be an extension of the lesion into the right orbit with a possible mucocele.

b) (i) Rhinosinusitis (acute on chronic or recurrent); (ii) Fungal sinusitis (iii) Dental abscess with secondary sinusitis (iv) Neoplastic lesion

c) Bent & Kuhn diagnostic criteria

   i. 5 major

      1. Atopy (on history or serology to fungal antigen or allergy testing)
      2. Nasal polyposis
      3. Characteristic CT scan findings (double density sign)
      4. Positive fungal smear
      5. Allergic mucin

   ii. 6 minor

      1. Asthma
      2. Unilateral predominance
      3. Bone erosion on radiography
      4. Fungal culture
      5. Charcot-Leyden crystals
      6. Eosinophilia

d) Invasive vs non-invasive

e) Some RCT's have shown benefit

2.11 A special nasal deformity

A 24-year old lady presents to clinic with an abnormal looking nose. There is no history of trauma and she also complains of nasal crusting and recurrent epistaxis. The photo below shows her nose shortly before undergoing an examination under anaesthesia (EUA).

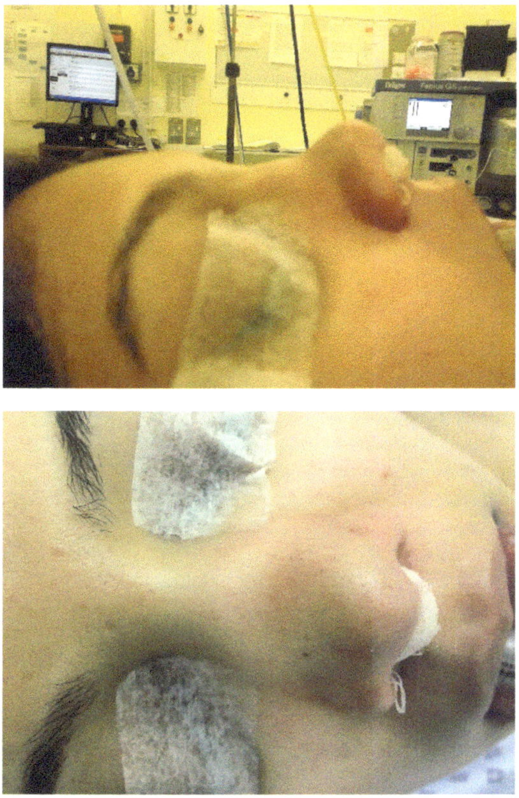

Questions

a) What is the abnormality depicted in the photo?

b) List five differentials for this finding

c) The patient presents at a later date in renal failure – a cANCA immunofluorescent pattern due to antibody reactivity against the leukocyte proteinase-3 protein (PR3) is found to be positive – what is the diagnosis?

d) List 5 symptoms that the patient may experience

e) List 4 ENT-related signs that the patient may have

f) What 4 investigations would you like to perform?

Answers

a) Saddle nose deformity

b) Trauma, Wegener's granulomatosis, sarcoidosis, cocaine abuse, previous nasal/septal surgery

c) Wegener's granulomatosis (a systemic vasculitis now known as 'Granulomatosis with polyangitis' – GPA – due to Wegener's Nazi affiliations)

d) Haemoptysis, cough, dyspnoea, haematuria, fever/night sweats, arthralgia/myalgia, cutaneous lesions, hearing loss

e) Epistaxis, nasal obstruction, rhinosinusitis, septal ulceration/perforation, subglottic stenosis, middle ear effusion with associated conductive hearing loss – may have SNHL too

f) (i) Nasal biopsy for histology and culture; (ii) Imaging guided by clinical signs; (iii) cANCA, ANA, Rheumatoid Factor plus serum ACE; (iv) CXR; (v) Urinalysis

2.12 An unusual nose

This 60-year old man is referred to you with longstanding change in the appearance of his nose

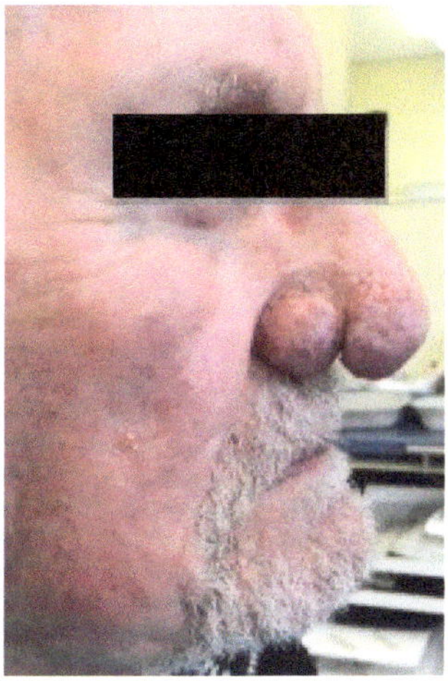

Questions

a) What is the diagnosis?

b) What is this condition associated with?

c) Name an investigation that may be useful for this patient?

d) What other specialist input may be helpful?

e) What are the treatment options? List 4

Answers

a) Rhinophyma – thickened sebaceous skin and enlarged pores

b) Even though aetiology is unknown, it is associated with acne rosacea. There is no link with excess alcohol intake.

c) Punch biopsy to exclude BCC/SCC

d) Dermatologist for management of concomitant skin disease and psychologist support for any mental health problems concerning body image

e) Preventative therapy (cleansing skin with defatting agents, anti inflammatory agents, antibiotics, benzoyl peroxidase lotions and isotretinoin)

   Surgery for treatment of surgical deformity (partial or full thickness excision using laser, dermabrasion, scalpel, microdebrider)

2.13 A 'runny' nose

This 39 year old business woman presents with right sided watery nasal discharge. There is no history of trauma or previous surgery. She did not mention any nasal blockage, itching sneezing, pain, headache, pressure symptoms or anosmia.

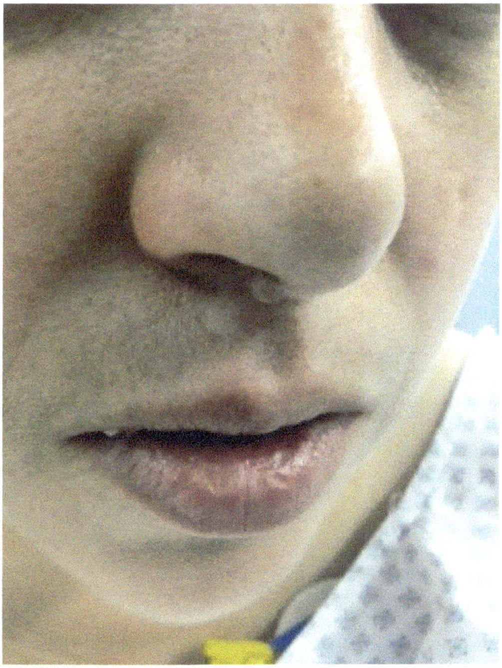

Questions

a) List 2 differential diagnoses?

b) Which simple test can be done in the clinic to assist with the diagnosis?

c) Which other test would you request to help confirm the diagnosis?

d) What imaging studies would you request?

e) List 3 ways of checking for raised intracranial pressure

Answers

a) Vasomotor Rhinitis and CSF rhinorrhoea

b) Dipstick the fluid for glucose

c) Beta-2 transferrin on collected fluid

d) CT skull base and T2-weighted MRI

e) Fundoscopy, lumbar puncture and ocular ultrasound (measurement of the optic nerve sheath diameter)

CHAPTER 3

Otology

3.1 Recurrent ear infections in a healthy young man

A 25 year old swimmer comes to clinic with a history of recurrent ear infections. On otoscopy you see the following:

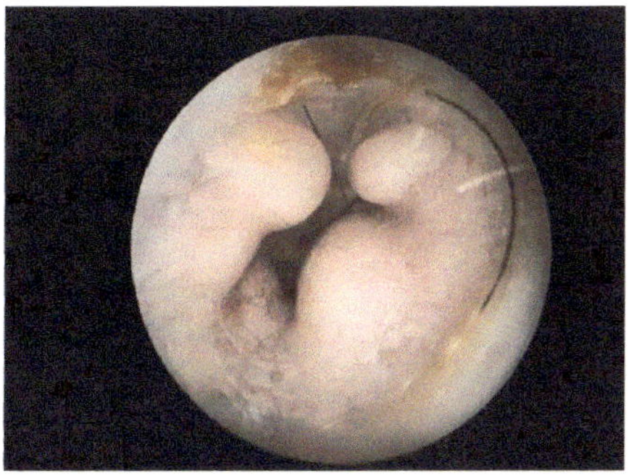

Questions

a) Describe the picture

b) Which part of the temporal bone is associated with these lesions?

c) What is the proposed aetiological factor for this condition?

d) List two treatment options for this patient?

e) What two structures are vulnerable at surgery?

Answers

a) Multiple lesions extending from the ear canal wall into the canal, causing obstruction – consistent with a diagnosis of canal exostoses

b) The tympanic ring

c) Exposure to cold water and wind (eg swimmers)

d) (i) **Conservative** (avoid water, use ear plug) and (ii) **Surgical** removal of exostoses with drill.

e) TMJ and Facial nerve (hence the importance to perform a CT scan before canaloplasty)

3.2 Discharging ear

The photo below is of the left ear

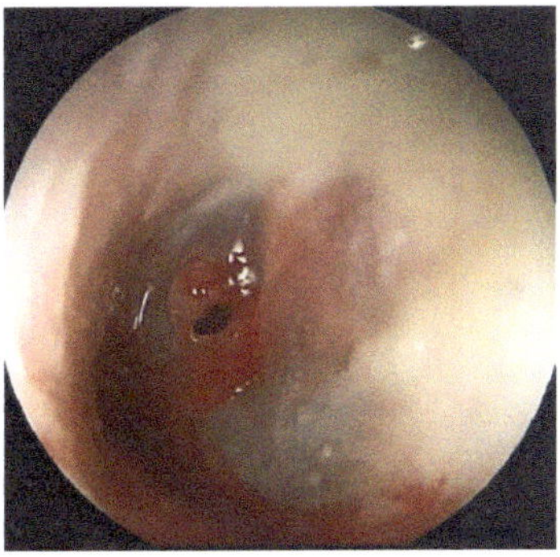

Questions

a) Describe the picture

b) What complications may arise if this condition is left untreated? List 3

c) What simple measures can be undertaken to reduce risk of infections? List 2

d) What surgical procedures may have been performed on this patient previously? List 2

e) What are the options for treatment? List 3

f) In the context of a maximal conductive hearing loss deficit, what other otological procedure should be considered?

Answers

a) Left ear endoscopic view showing an antero- inferior central perforation, with associated pus and blood in the ear canal

b) Recurrent infections may lead to scarring of the tympanic membrane (ie tympanosclerosis) and subsequent fibrosis and fixation of the ossicles causing a conductive hearing loss. Recurrent infections may also give rise to SNHL as a result of ototoxic secretions from infective organisms

c) Water protection (Vaseline + cotton wool), treatment of infections

d) Grommet insertion and tympanoplasty

e) Conservative (water protection), Medical (topical antibiotics), Surgical (myringoplasty)

f) Ossiculoplasty

3.3 A 'sucked-in' tympanic membrane

This photo is from a 28 year old man who presents to clinic with hearing loss. PTA reveals a conductive hearing loss with an air-bone gap of 30dBHL on the left. Tympanometry gives a Type 'C' curve.

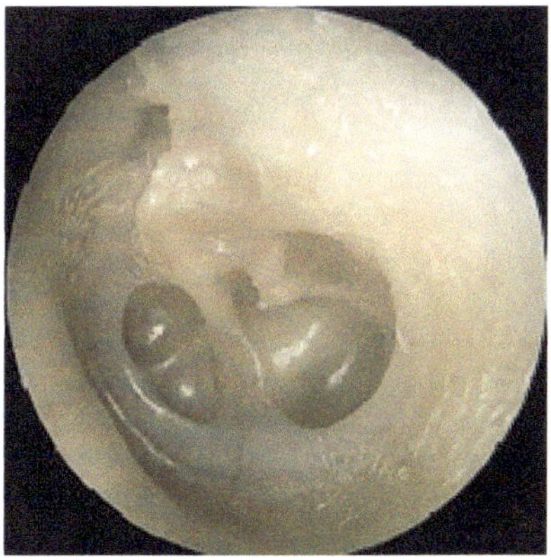

Questions

a) Describe the image

b) How is this condition graded?

c) List 2 risks of associated with this condition?

d) What underlying condition is thought to play a role?

e) List 4 important aspects of this patient's management

f) Describe the structure + embryology of the tympanic membrane

Answers

a) Endoscopic view of a left tympanic membrane with

retractions of the *pars tensa* and *pars flaccida*. The incudostapedial joint is clearly visible.

b) Sade classification for *pars tensa* retraction, Tos classification for *pars flaccida* retraction

c) Erosion of the ossicles (leading to maximum conductive hearing loss of 60dB), Development of cholesteatoma and associated infection

d) Eustachian tube dysfunction

e) Close observation, scrupulous aural toilet, keep ear dry. Improvement of middle ear ventilation (eg Valsalva manoeuvres, ventilation devices, treat underlying rhinitis / post-nasal space oedema)

f) Outer layer – squamous (ectoderm, first branchial cleft), middle layer - fibrous (mesoderm), inner layer mucosal (endoderm, first branchial pouch)

3.4 Chronically discharging ear

The image shows a left tympanic membrane with attic cholesteatoma

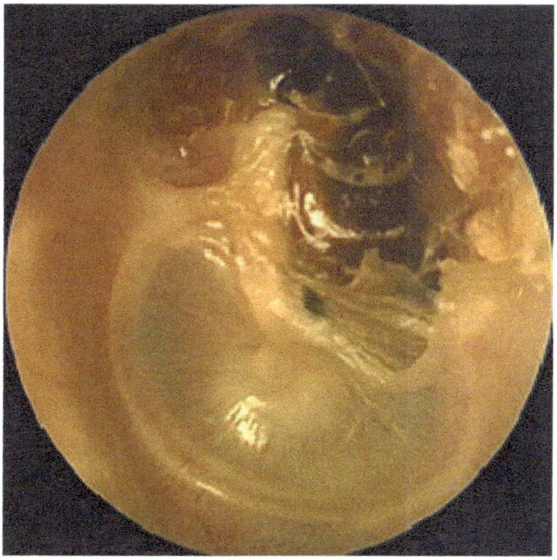

Questions

a) What is cholesteatoma?

b) How is it classified?

c) How can complications be classified?

d) List two of each type of classification

e) What imaging modality other than CT is useful in planning operative management?

Answers

a) Keratinizing squamous epithelium in the middle ear cleft leading to bone and soft tissue erosion and infection

b) Primary acquired (retraction pocket, negative middle ear pressure), secondary acquired (perforation, trauma or iatrogenic), congenital (embryonic epithelial rest cells (Michael's body).

c) Otologic, extracranial, Intracranial

d)

i. Otologic – Destruction of ossicular chain, hearing loss, perilymph fistula, facial nerve palsy, acute mastoiditis, Gradenigo syndrome

ii. Extracranial – Bezold abscess (Sternocleidomastoid), Citelli abscess (digastric), Lucs abscess (temporalis)

iii. Intracranial complications – Meningitis, extradural/subdural abscess, intracerebral abscess, encephalitis, lateral/sigmoid sinus thrombosis, hydrocephalus

e) Diffusion weighted MRI – can distinguish between cholesteatoma and inflammatory tissue

3.5 Traumatic hearing loss

A 40 year old is knocked off his bicycle. After clearing his head and c-spine he is noted to have a profound hearing loss on the right side and bleeding from his ear canal. A CT of the head is performed that shows a fracture of the temporal bone.

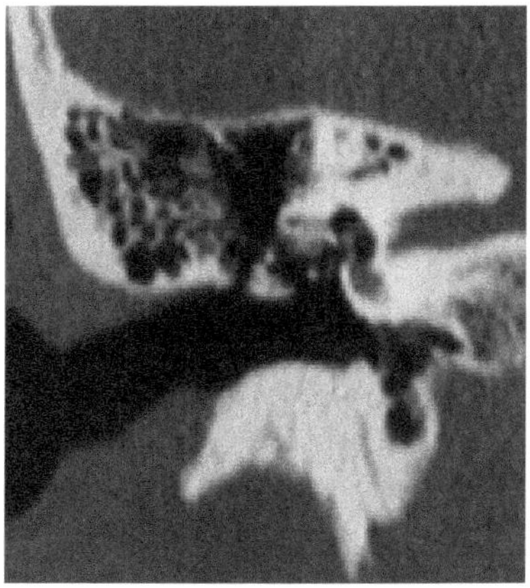

Questions

a) What type of fracture does the CT show?

b) What two types of fracture are encountered clinically and what is their preponderance?

c) What other clinical findings are sometimes present? List 3

d) What two further investigations might you arrange?

e) How would you determine the nature of clear exudate from the ear canal?

f) If there is an acute facial palsy, what type of fracture is more likely

Answers

a) Longitudinal temporal bone fracture

b) Longitudinal (75%) and Transverse (25%)

c) Haemotympanum, facial palsy, CSF otorrhoea

d) PTA and Angiogram if carotid injury likely

e) Beta-2-transferrin is only found in CSF and endolymph and therefore may be of diagnostic value

f) Transverse

3.6 An interesting tympanic membrane

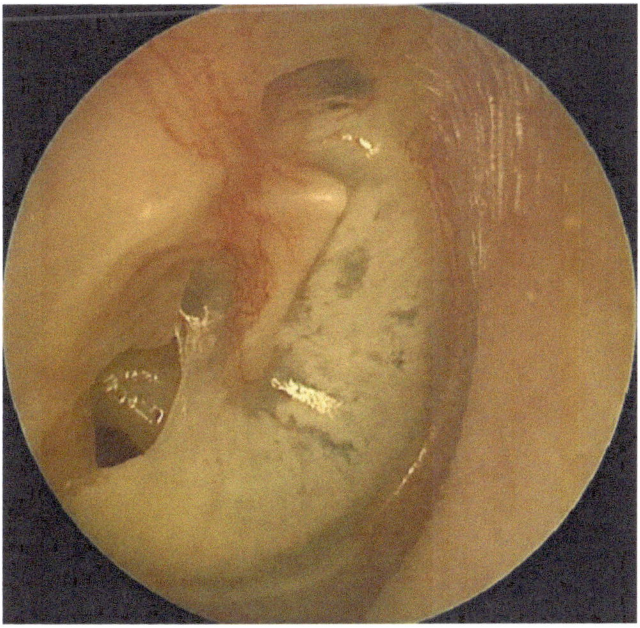

Questions

a) Which ear is shown in photograph above?

b) List 2 abnormalities show in the photograph

c) What graft may be used to repair the ear drum. List 3

d) Name three surgical approaches to close the defect

e) What techniques can be used for graft placement? List 2

f) What is the maximum conductive hearing loss possible?

g) Is this patient likely to have a significant hearing loss compared with someone with a defect anteriorly?

Answers

a) Right ear

b) (i) Tympanosclerosis affecting the pars tensa mainly and (ii) a posterior peforation adjacent to the round window

c) Temporalis fascia, tragal perichondrium, tragal cartilage

d) Permeatal, post-auricular, end-aural

e) Medial (underlay) technique and lateral (overlay) technique

f) 60dB

g) Yes, because of the baffle effect (sound entering the inner ear via both the oval and round window)

3.7 An eye, ear and balance problem

A 35-year-old presents to clinic with a 6-month history of lacrimation and photophobia. He currently has been experiencing episodic vertigo and associated hearing loss and tinnitus.

Questions

a) What is the most likely diagnosis?

b) What is believed to be the underlying pathophysiology?

c) What is the eye condition called in this disease?

d) What type of hearing loss will this patient have?

e) How can this condition be treated? List 2 treatment options

f) List 3 other autoimmune conditions that may affect hearing and balance

Answers

a) Cogan syndrome

b) Unknown but believed to be an autoimmune reaction leading to hydrops, similar to Meniere's

c) Non syphilitic interstitial keratitis (blurriness initially that can rapidly progress to blindness)

d) Typically a sensorineural hearing loss

e) High-dose oral corticosteroids (usually resolves hearing and vestibular dysfunction). Can consider cyclophosphamide or azathioprine

f) Polyarteritis nodosa, Wegener's granulomatosis (GPA), relapsing polychondritis, systemic lupus erythematosus.

3.8 A hearing device

A patient with hearing loss has the following prosthesis attached to her head:

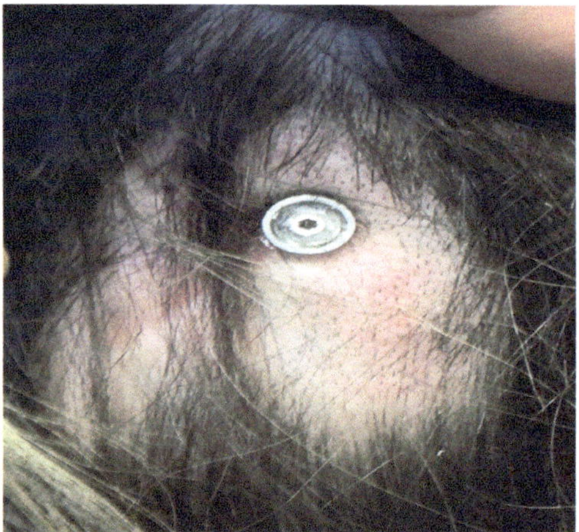

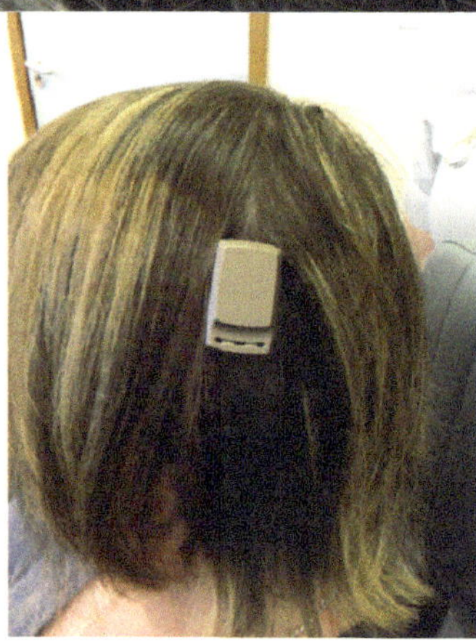

Questions

a) What is this device?

b) What kind of hearing loss is this most suited to?

c) Name three indications for this device

d) What are its main components?

e) Name a syndrome in which this might be of use

f) Why might someone with a profound unilateral hearing loss benefit from this device?

g) Name two potential complications of this device

h) What alternative and newer devices may be considered in such cases?

Answer

a) Abutment for a Bone Anchored Hearing Aid (BAHA) and a fitted processor

b) Conductive hearing loss

c) Patients with hearing loss, unable to benefit from an air conduction hearing aid due to a persistently discharging ear, canal stenosis or microtia, also single sided deafness.

d) A vibrating sound processor that is coupled to a titanium fixture/abutment that is surgically implanted into the skull

e) Treacher-Collins (craniofacial abnormalities including canal atresia), Goldenhaar syndrome

f) Reduces the head shadow effect

g) Soft tissue overgrowth, infection and pain. The implanted titanium screw can also come out especially if angled insertion or poor quality bone

h) The use of abutment free devices (e.g. 'Bonebridge' or 'BAHA Attract') allowing coupling through magnets

3.9 A bionic ear

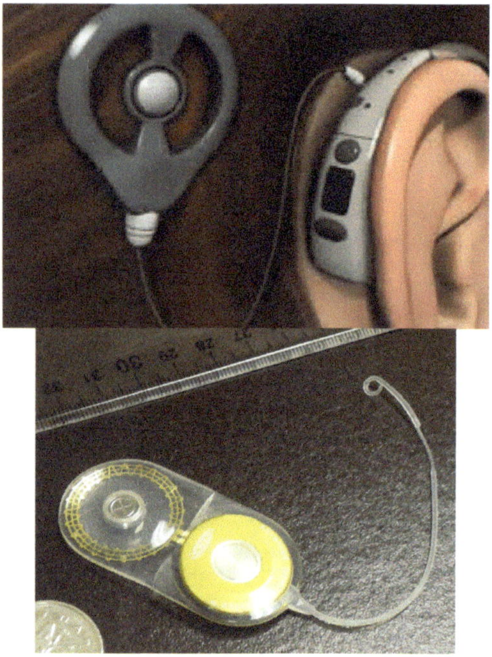

Questions

a) What is this device?

b) List the 3 main components

c) What two groups are candidates for the device?

d) What is electro-acoustic stimulation?

e) List 4 contra-indications for inserting this device.

Answers

a) Cochlear implant

b) Receiver, processor, implant with electrode

c) (i) Pre-lingual deaf children (offered simultaneous bilateral implants) (ii) Post-lingual deaf children or adults (single implants unless blind or had meningitis).

d) The process of stimulating the cochlea with both electrical stimulation via the implanted electrode and also by an acoustic hearing aid via separate devices or by a hybrid processor

e) Absolute contraindication is abscent cochlea (Michel deformity). Relative contraindications: Infected ear, OME, retrocochlear disease, expected non-compliance with extensive rehabilitation program, temporal bone fracture involving otic capsule

3.10 A middle ear lesion

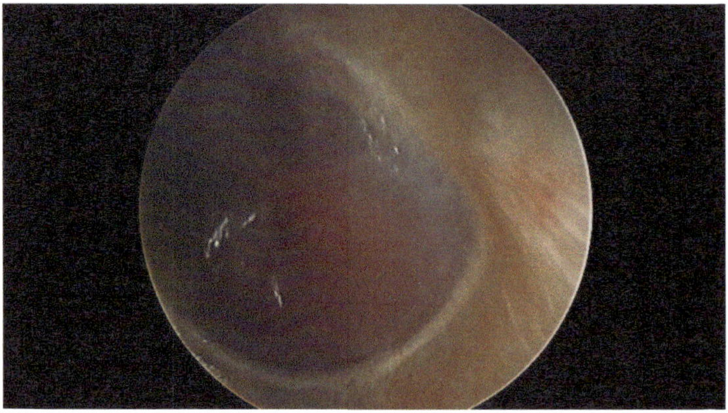

Questions

a) Describe the image

b) What is the most likely diagnosis? List 2 other differentials

c) Assuming this is a neoplastic lesion, what is the embryological basis?

d) What is the main blood supply?

e) What symptoms may this patient present with? List 4

f) Name two clinical signs that may be elicited in this condition

g) What treatment options are available?

h) What investigation (excluding imaging) is essential in the work-up to definitive treatment?

Answers:

a) Otoscopic photograph of a left tympanic membrane with a pink lesion occupying the lower middle ear space.

b) Glomus tumour (glomus tympanicum if it is confined to the middle ear). Otospongiosis and high jugular bulb

c) Neuroendocrine neoplasm arising from neural crest cells of the parasympathetic nerves

d) Ascending pharyngeal artery

e) Pulsatile tinnitus, local erosive effects – Otalgia, hearing loss, vertigo, facial palsy

f) Brown's sign (blanching of the tumour on pneumatic otoscopy) and Aquino's sign (cessation of tumour pulsation with occlusion of the ipsilateral carotid artery)

g) Conservative (wait and watch), Surgical excision with or without embolization of feeding blood vessel(s).

h) Urinary catecholamines (adrenaline and noradrenaline) and their metabolites (vanillylmandelic acid, VMA) in a 24 hour collection

3.11 A swollen ear

This child is referred with a grossly swollen ear following a clash of heads on a bouncy castle.

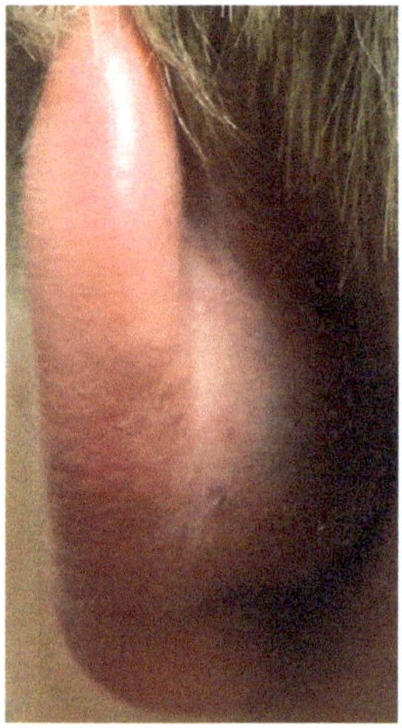

Questions

a) What is the likely diagnosis?

b) What are the risks of leaving this condition untreated?

c) What is the anatomical basis of this?

d) How will you treat this. Give 2 options

e) What follow-up is needed?

Answers

a) Pinna haematoma

b) Ear deformity (i.e. cauliflower ear) due to chondritis +/- abscess formation that eventually leads to scarring of the pinna due to avascular necrosis

c) The auricular cartilage derives its blood supply from its perichondrium. Thus, a haematoma that forms between the perichondrium and cartilage, deprives it from a blood supply

d) If small and first attempt, aspiration with a large bore needle followed by a compressive dressing. If large or re-collection of haematoma, incision and drainage is the treatment of choice. A 'through and through' suturing of a dental roll can be used as a compressive dressing for either treatment

e) Oral antibiotics, removal of the sutures in 5 days +/- re-evacuation of the haematoma

3.12 A prosthesis for rehabilitation of hearing loss

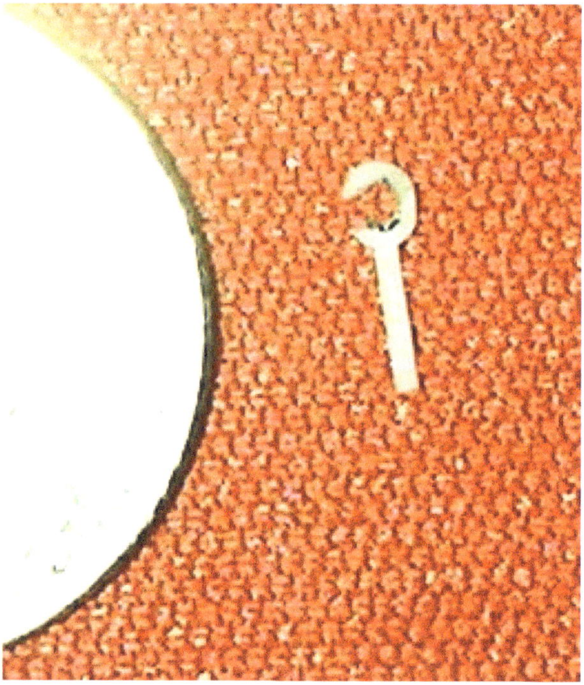

Questions

a) What is shown in this picture?

b) What surgical procedure would this be used in?

c) List 3 absolute contra-indications of this procedure

d) List 6 risks associated with this procedure

e) What is the relative importance of the diagnosis of Menieres disease when performing this procedure?

Answers

a) A fluoroplastic stapes piston

b) Stapedectomy

c) Active ear (infection); pregnancy; tinnitus as the sole symptom

d) Infection (including meningitis), bleeding, hearing loss/dead ear, vertigo, facial nerve injury, damage to chorda tympani, perforation of tympanic membrane, displacement of prosthesis, need for further surgery, failure of insertion of prosthesis

e) Increased risk of dead ear due to increase in size of saccule and closer proximity to footplate

3.13 Anatomy of the pinna

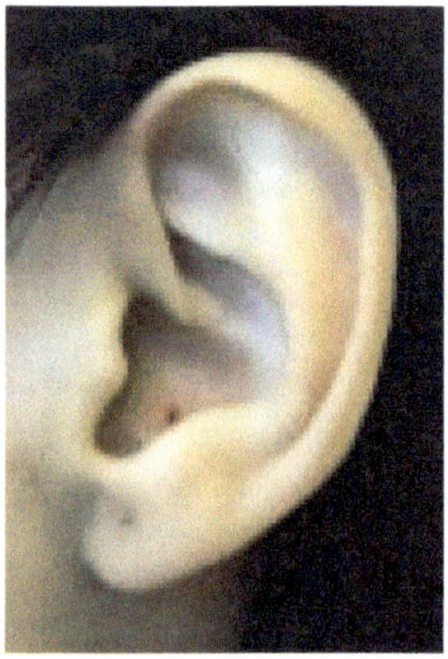

Questions

On the ear above, identify the following:

a) Anti-helix

b) Superior crus of anti-helix

c) Inferior crus of anti-helix

d) Concha cymba

e) Concha cavum

f) Tragus

g) Anti-tragus

h) Inter-tragal notch

i) Triangularis fossa

j) Scapha

k) Lobule

l) Helix

m) helical crus

n) external ear meatus

Answers

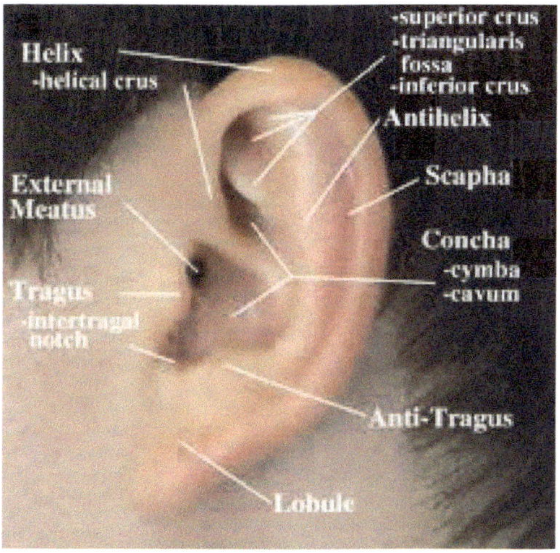

3.14 Noise in the ear

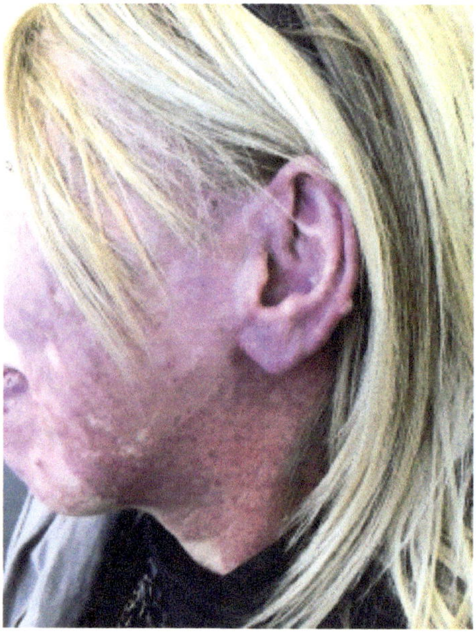

Questions

a) What does the photo show?

b) What type of noise would you suspect in her head?

c) List 4 relevant investigations

d) What are the two main modalities of treatment?

e) Are there any useful medicines to treat tinnitus? List 3

f) What is tinnitology?

Answers

a) Port wine stain

b) Pulsatile tinnitus

c) PTA and tympanograms, carotid Doppler, MRI/MRA, CT temporal bone, optic nerve sheath diameter to assess intracranial pressure

d) Noise therapy (eg white noise masker) and behavioural therapy

e) Yes. Benzodiazepines, antidepressants and dexamethasone

f) The study of how the perception of an aberrant auditory phenomenon can be translated into sensation and effect.

3.15 Skull base anatomy

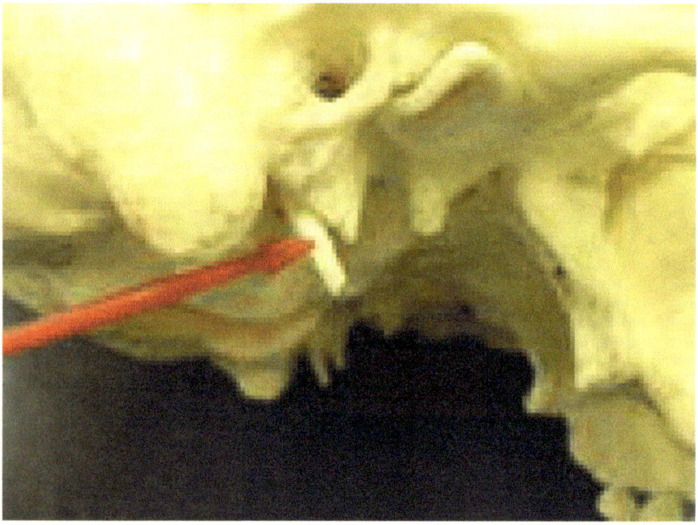

Questions

a) What structure is the arrow pointing at?

b) List all the attachments of that bony projection

c) Name the nerve supply to each muscle listed in question 2

d) Which syndrome is associated with calcification of this structure

Answers

a) Right styloid process of the temporal bone

b) 2 LIGAMENTS: stylohyoid and stylomandibular

3 MUSCLES: styloglossus, stylohyoid and stylopharyngeus

c) Styloglossus – hypoglossal nerve (CN XII)

Stylohyoid – facial nerve (CN VII)

Stylopharyngeus – glossopharyngeal nerve.

e) Eagle's syndrome

3.16 An odd tympanic membrane

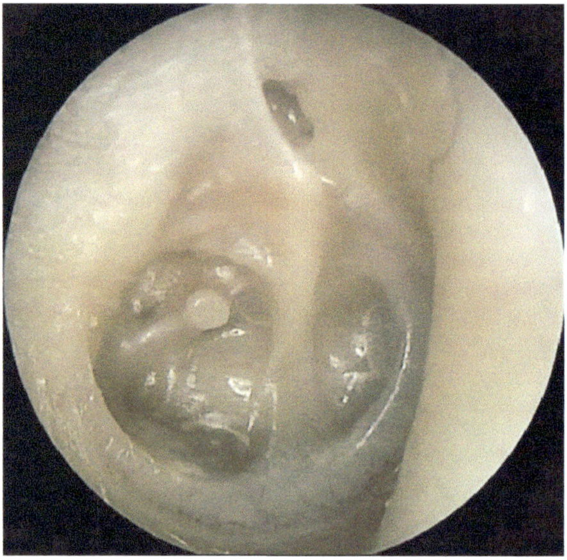

Questions

a) Which ear is this?

b) List 4 otoscopic findings

c) What is the diagnosis?

d) What are the treatment options?

e) In the presence of attic cholesteatoma what would your surgical options be?

f) List 5 factors that you would take into account when deciding the most appropriate management option for this patient?

Answers

a) Right ear

b) Ear canal: normal

   i. Tympanic membrane: Tos Grade 1-2 retraction of pars flaccida. No erosion of attic wall. Sade grade 3-4 retraction of pars tensa (touching onto promontory and if adherent to it then grade 4)

   ii. Ossicles: Medialised malleus. Only stapes head is seen; long process of incus and incudostapedial joint eroded.

   iii. No presence of cholesteatoma/squamous debri

c) Chronic inactive squamous otitis media leading to adhesive otitis media. (NB. try to avoid using the term chronic suppurative or non-suppurative otitis media)

d) Conservative

   i. Wait and watch

   ii. Hearing aid

   Surgical

   i. Ventilation tube (grommet; mini-grommet; extra-annular t-tube)

   ii. Tympanoplasty (with resection of retracted drum segment and reconstruction of neo-tympanic membrane) +/- ossiculoplasty

e) Atticotomy, modified radical mastoidectomy or

combined approach tympanoplasty

f) Patient wishes, age of patient, hearing of affected ear, state of affected ear (i.e. presence/absence of cholesteatoma; presence/absence of infection), hearing and state of opposite ear, patient general health – presence of co-morbidities

3.17 An under-developed ear

This 30-year old man has abnormal ears

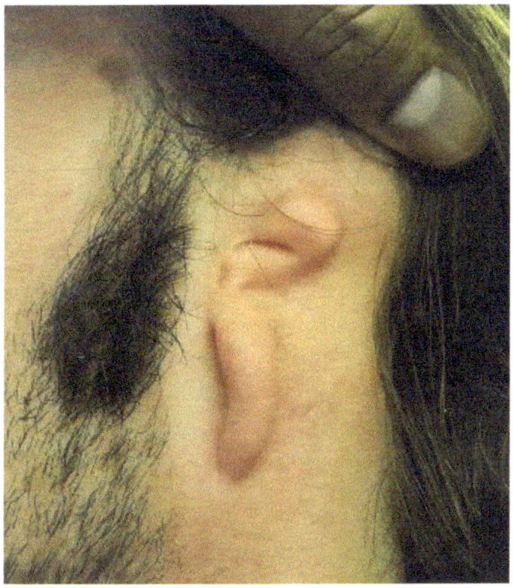

Questions

a) What is the name of this condition?

b) How is it commonly classified?

c) What are the issues associated with this condition? List 3

d) How would you manage this? List 3

e) What factors should be considered if surgery is to be undertaken. List 2

Answers

a) Microtia

b) Grade 1-4

1. Small pinna, normal anatomy
2. Some abnormality of the pinna, canal patent, closed or partially closed
3. Pinna remnant only, canal absent
4. Complete absence of pinna and canal (anotia)

c) Functional

   i. CHL up to 60dBHL due to canal atresia +/- ossicular dysfunction

   ii. Inability to wear glasses

   Cosmetic

   iii. Psychological effects

d)

   i. Management of the hearing: BAHA on a softband / full BAHA for CHL

   ii. Management of the external ear deformity: Surgical reconstruction or prosthesis

   iii. Psychologist input if appropriate

e)

   i. Timing of surgery is crucial. Ideally the patient should be fully involved in the decision making

   ii. Imaging of the temporal bone for further evaluation of the hearing loss. May also be used when considering a prosthetic ear (surgical planning)

   iii. Multidisciplinary team involvement

3.18 A "small" infection with hugely debilitating effects

You are asked to see an otherwise well 20-year-old male patient in the Emergency Department. He has presented with sudden onset severe vertigo, hearing loss and nystagmus (fast component towards the left). He has been severely sick and can hardly stand. Otoscopy is normal.

Questions

a) What is your most likely diagnosis

b) What is the most likely cause?

c) What investigations would you consider? List 3

d) How would you manage this patient? List 3 aspects of your management

e) During your assessment, the patient confides in you about a 'lesion' he has just noted over his penis. How might this be relative to this case?

Answers

a) Acute left-sided labyrinthitis. Vestibular neuronitis is not the correct answer as this patient has experienced auditory and vestibular dysfunction.

b) Believed to be related to viral infection. Associated viruses include rubella, herpes simplex virus, reoviruses, cytomegalovirus, influenza and mumps

c) Most cases resolve spontaneously so investigations in the acute setting are limited. Would consider routine bloods (if suspected inflammatory component) and an audiogram and tympanogram (to confirm sensorineural hearing loss and exclude any effusion respectively). In the presence of any neurology or persistent symptoms an MRI would be needed to exclude a central cause or an acoustic neuroma. Finally, Electronystagmography (ENG) and calorics can be performed if symptoms persist.

d) (i) In acute setting a limited course of vestibular suppression (prochlorperazine oral, intramuscular or buccal); (ii) Because of hearing loss (if possible confirmed with audiogram or at least clinically) should consider oral steroids; (iii) Intravenous fluids need to be considered if unable to tolerate anything orally; (iv) Patient should try to start activities early; (v) Vestibular rehabilitation exercises (Cawthorne Cooksey) should be provided

e) This is a syphilitic chancre signifying luetic labyrinthitis caused by *Treponema pallidum*. May occur in primary, secondary or tertiary syphilis.

3.19 Bilateral hearing loss

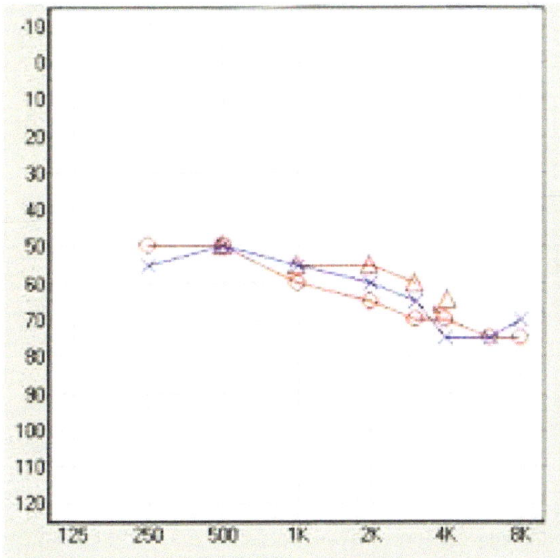

This is the pure tone audiogram of a 15 year old man who has recently underwent surgery to remove a large ependymoma from his spinal cord.

Questions

a) What is the most likely underlying condition?

b) Which gene is involved in this condition?

c) What is the mode of inheritance of this condition?

d) Which device is available to rehabilitate the hearing loss?

e) What treatment options exist? List 3

Answers

a) Bilateral acoustic neuromas associated Neurofibromatosis Type II

b) The gene involved is a tumour suppressor on chromosome 22 (Ch 22q11) and encodes a peptide product called 'Merlin' (aka schwannomin, neurofibromin 2

c) The inherited version of the disease is an autosomal dominant disorder (Mendelian inheritance). Half of cases however are due to a spontaneous (i.e. de novo) mutation

d) Initially an air conduction hearing aid should be used. If surgery is done for the lesions then brainstem implants may be inserted at the same time.

e) Conservative with serial MRIs

   Medical: Stereotactic radiation +/- Bevacizumab (Avastin, VEGF antagonist)

   Surgery

3.20 A pink tympanic membrane

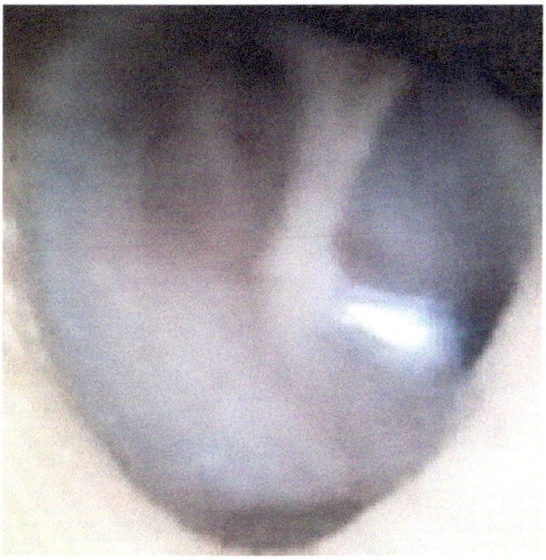

This is the right tympanic membrane of a patient complaining of hearing loss. Her sister had the same problem and had a successful operation to rehabilitate the associated hearing loss.

Questions

a) What is the most likely diagnosis?

b) What pathological process defines this condition?

c) What is Paracusis of Willisi?

d) What does the 2kHz drop on the audiogram represent?

e) List 5 management options

f) What do you understand by the term overclosure of the air-bone gap?

Answers

a) Otosclerosis (*Schwartz's sign* is present in the posterior segment of the tympanic membrane, ie, the drum has a flamingo pink blush due to increased blood supply to the otospongiotic focus

b) The replacement of mature lamellar bone by woven bone that has greater cellularity and vascularity

c) Paracusis willisi is a finding in otosclerosis whereby hearing is better in the presence of background noise.

d) Carhart notch (the 2kHz drop) is considered an artefact of bone conduction due to the fact that the ossicular chain vibrates at its maximum in this frequency

e) Conservative: Wait and watch/reassurance

   Medical: Hearing aids, bone anchored hearing aids, fluoride

   Surgical: Stapedectomy

f) Overclosure refers to the better post-operative hearing (air-conduction) compared to the pre-operative bone conduction thresholds. This can be explained by the artefact of the Carhart notch

3.21 Otoacoustic emissions (sky above the fence)

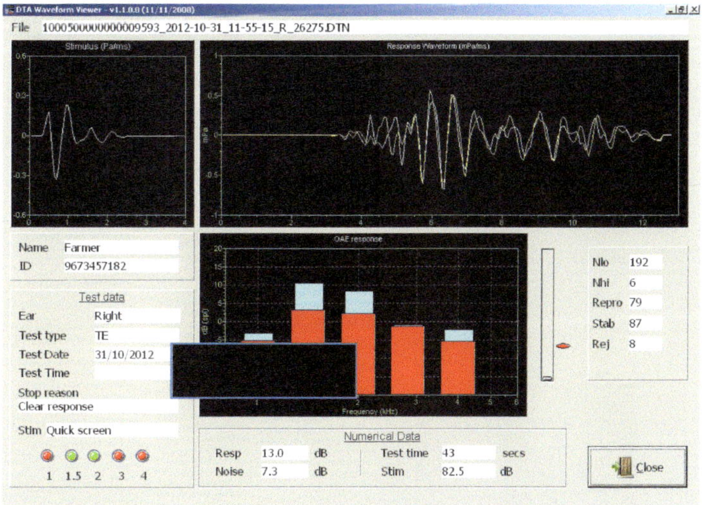

Questions

a) What is the name of the graph shown above?

b) Which components of the inner ear are responsible for the graph?

c) What is the main use of this investigation?

d) Name one other use of this test.

e) List 3 elements that are important for interpretation of the graph

f) Is this investigation useful for retrocochlear disorders such as acoustic neuromas?

Answers

a) Transient evoked otoacoustic emission graph

b) Outer hair cells

c) Universal neonatal screening programme (main aim is to identify congenital hearing loss greater than 40dB)

d) Non-organic hearing loss

e) Stimulus, probe stability and signal to noise ratio (but note that 2 or more green lights on the bottom left hand corner indicate PASS or 'clear response')

f) No. It only provides useful information about cochlear and middle ear functions.

3.22 A weird but important waveform

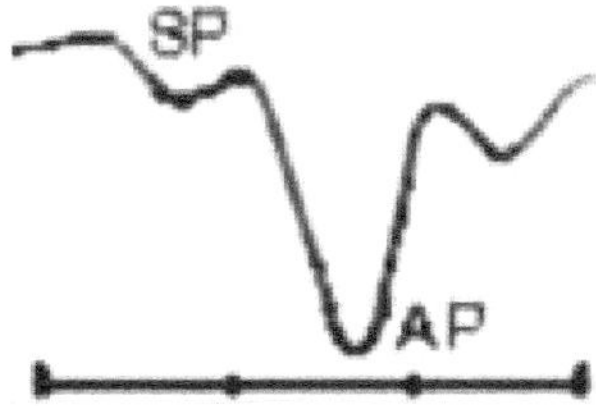

Questions

a) What does electrocochleography measure?

b) What does the wave consist of?

c) List 2 clinical applications for its use

d) What electrodes are required in order to perform the procedure?

e) What measures are pathognomonic for Meniere's disease?

Answers

a) It measures the electrical output of the cochlea and the auditory nerve in response to an auditory stimulus

b) The cochlear microphonic (CM): indicates cochlear hair cells are intact

The summating potential (SP): represents an alteration of the electrical potential baseline in response to an auditory stimulus

The action potential (AP): it is the electrical response of the auditory nerve and it is useful for determining thresholds

c) Threshold determination

   Meniere's disease diagnosis

   Intra-operative monitoring with certain diseases

d) Ground electrode: Placed on forehead

   Reference electrode: On mastoid prominence of tested ear

   Active electrode: Can be extratympanic or transtympanic

e) Increased SP/AP ratio (>30%)

CHAPTER 4

Head and neck

4.1 Painless facial swelling

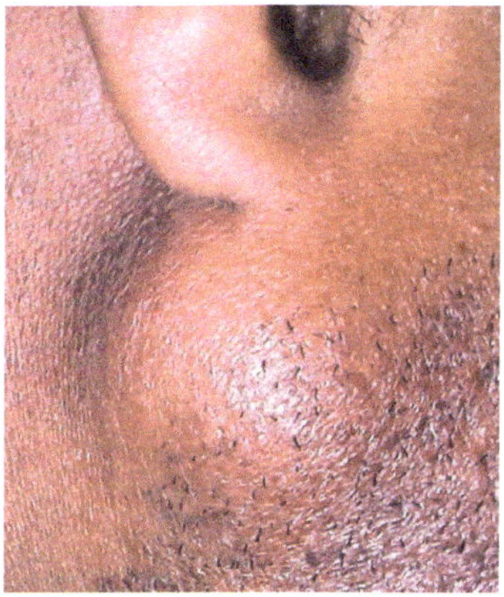

This 40 year old man presents to clinic with a painless right-sided facial swelling that has grown over several years.

Questions

a) Describe this lesion

b) What is the most likely diagnosis?

c) What other features might be present in this patient? List 4

d) What is the gold standard diagnostic procedures?

e) With the diagnosis confirmed, what course of action would you propose and why?

f) What would you counsel the patient for when taking consent for an operation?

g) What is the risk of recurrence?

Answers

a) A mass over the angle of the jaw, probably arising from the tail of the parotid gland

b) Pleomorphic adenoma

c) Facial palsy, intra-oral swelling (deep lobe involvement in 10% of cases), Dysphagia (rare, unless pharyngeal extension), shortness of breath or hoarseness (if laryngeal involvement)

d) US scan and FNAC

e) Surgical excision because there is a small risk of malignant transformation (and this cannot be excluded by FNA alone)

f) Facial nerve injury, Frey's syndrome, salivary fistula, seroma, loss of sensation of the ear lobe (greater auricular nerve), recurrence

g) Less than 4 percent

4.2 Approaching hoarseness

GP referral (2 week wait): Thank you for seeing this 50-year old patient with a two-month history of hoarseness.

Questions

a) List 10 things you would ask in the history

b) What medications may cause hoarseness? List 5

c) List 10 differentials

d) What would you include in your examination?

e) If you identified a suspicious lesion, what would you do next? List 3 things

Answers

a) Character of hoarseness: onset and duration, time course (acute vs chronic)

Associated symptoms: odynophagia, dysphagia, aspiration, weight loss, otalgia, heartburn

Contributing factors: recent cold, cough, congestion, vocal abuse,

Past medical history: general, previous laryngeal trauma, previous intubation, previous surgery or irradiation (e.g. neck surgery or any surgery close to RLNs)

Drug history

Social history: occupation, tobacco or alcohol

b) Warfarin and thrombolytics can cause vocal fold haematoma; bisphosphonates can cause chemical laryngitis; ACE inhibitors can cause a dry cough;

testosterone has a hormonal effect; antipsychotics may cause dystonia; inhaled steroids can lead to mucosal irritation and fungal laryngitis

c) Congenital (e.g. web); infectious (viral, bacterial or fungal); idiopathic (muscle tension disorders); trauma related (cysts, nodules, voice abuse, Reinke's oedema, granulomas, caustic injuries); neoplasia (malignant or benign); endocrine (e.g. hypothyroidism); neurologic (e.g. vocal fold paralysis; MS, tremor, stroke, myasthenia gravis); systemic (e.g. GORD, connective tissue disorder, psychogenic)

d) Head and neck examination; assessment of voice; visualisation of vocal cords (e.g. flexible nasendoscopy); in a voice clinic videostroboscopy can be used; neurological assessment if necessary

e) Arrange urgent imaging (CT/MRI) PRIOR to urgent endoscopic assessment (panendoscopy and microlaryngoscopy) for tissue diagnosis; urgent referral to head and neck MDT

4.3 Laryngeal tumour

Surgical specimen from a patient with T4 laryngeal cancer

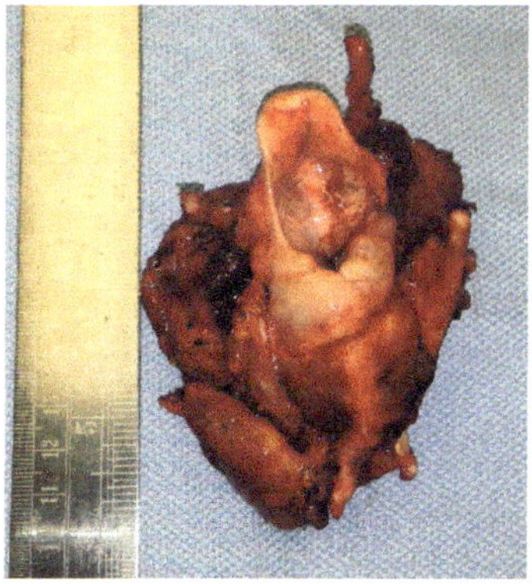

Questions

a) What type of histopathology is this patient most likely to have?

b) Which sites of the larynx can become involved? List commonest first and least common last

c) Why are laryngectomies performed less frequently now?

d) What factor can affect the speed of spread in patients with this disease?

e) List 6 complications associated with this procedure

f) What other procedure could be expected to be performed here?

g) List 3 options for a patient to regain speech following a laryngectomy

Answers

a) Squamous cell carcinoma (>95% of laryngeal cancer). Basaloid squamous cell carcinoma is a more aggressive high-grade variant

b) Glottis (50-75%), supraglottis (30-40%), subglottis (rare as primary site)

c) Chemoradiotherapy has become the treatment of choice for most cases, reserving laryngectomy for very advanced cases or relapsing disease (including salvage)

d) The presence (or absence) of lymphatics. Glottic tumours spread slower because of the lack of lymphatic drainage

e) Operative: bleeding, air embolism (IJV damage), pneumothorax, hypoglossal nerve damage

   Post-operative: haematoma, wound dehiscence (especially post radiotherapy), pharyngocutaneous fistula, chyle leak, skin necrosis,

   Late: Stomal recurrence, stomal stenosis, pharyngeal stricture, valve leak

f) Neck dissection

g) Tracheo-oesophageal puncture (TEP), oesophageal speech, electrolarynx

4.4 Difficulty swallowing

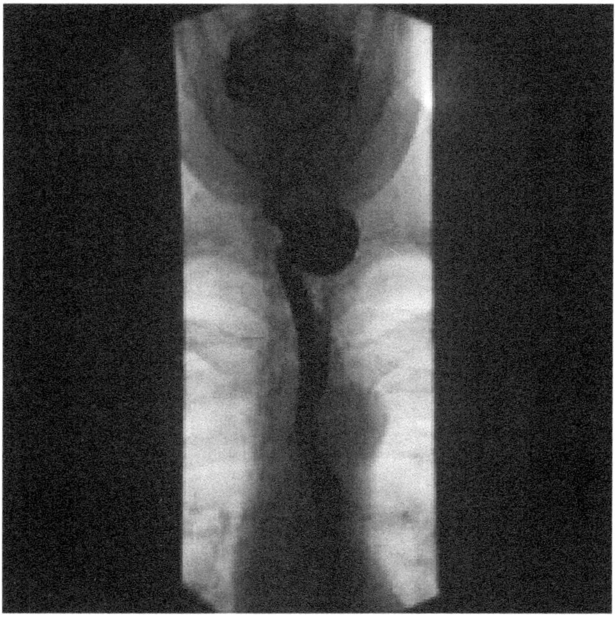

Questions

By looking at the investigation shown above, what is the most likely diagnosis?

a) What is the anatomical location of this defect?

b) How would you clinically assess such a patient? List 5 things

c) Should an endoscopic approach be used to treat this, what two bits of equipment would be needed?

d) What would you look out for in the immediate post-operative period in such a patient after endoscopic surgery? List 3 signs/symptoms

e) In a stable patient, what type of diet would you advise for the post-operative period?

Answers

a) Pharyngeal pouch (aka Zenker's diverticulum)

b) Killian's triangle. A triangular area of the posterior wall of the oesophagus that is considered weak, and is limited inferiorly by the cricopharyngeal and superiorly by the thyropharyngeal fibres of the inferior constrictor muscle

c) History: ask about weight loss, regurgitation (undigested food typically), malodorous breath, aspiration-like symptoms such as choking and coughing, pain.

   Examination: Full head and neck exam and flexible laryngoscopy. Purpose is to exclude any other diagnosis.

   Imaging: done already (Barium swallow)

d) A Weerda diverticuloscope and an endoscopic stapling gun for a pharyngeal pouch

e) Ensure no chest pain, surgical emphysema or tachycardia

f) Free fluids on the day of surgery followed by a soft diet the following day

4.5 Oral lesion

This lesion was found in the upper pole of the right tonsillar fossa. The lesion is two centimetres in length and has a 'mulberry' like appearance.

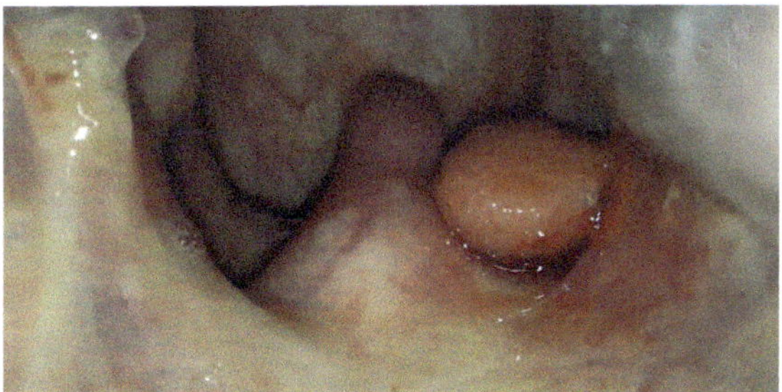

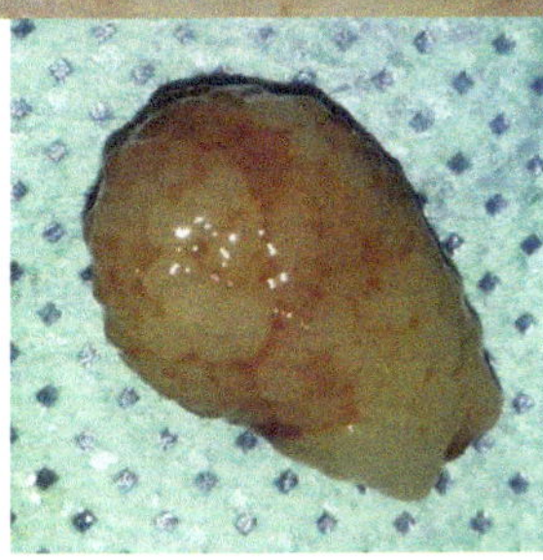

Questions

a) What is the likely diagnosis?

b) What is the most likely aetiology of this condition?

c) Which types of the causative organism are likely to be to blame?

d) What recent development should see a decrease in the incidence of this condition

e) Which population are still at risk despite this new development?

Answers

a) Oropharyngeal papilloma

b) Human papilloma virus (HPV)

c) HPV types 16 and 18

d) Introduction of vaccination programme in females

e) Males as the vaccine is currently only offered to females

4.6 Tracheostomy tubes

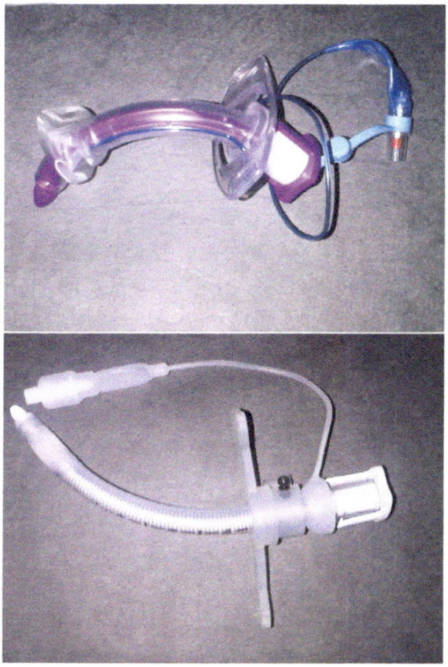

Questions

a) Name the tubes illustrated above and List 4 indications for a tracheostomy

b) What complications would you put on the consent form for this procedure? List 8

c) List 8 important aspects of post-tracheostomy care

d) What is a Passy-Muir?

e) List the principal steps of decannulation

Answers

a) Cuffed portex tube and cuffed Bivona extendable flange tube

   1. Bypass an obstruction (e.g. tumour)
   2. Avoid complications of prolonged intubation (e.g. ulcerations, granulations) and allow mechanical ventilation long-term
   3. Assist with trachea-bronchial suctioning (need for regular pulmonary toilet)
   4. Provide protection from aspiration
   5. Eliminate dead space (e.g. promote weaning from ventilator)

b) Bleeding, infection, subcutaneous emphysema, pneumothorax, trachea-oesophageal fistula formation, recurrent laryngeal nerve palsy, airway narrowing, tube dislodgement, tube obstruction, trachea-cutaneous fistula, death (in rare cases)

c)

   1. Prevent tube dislodgement in first few days (tube should be sutured to neck skin and have tightly placed tracheostomy tube ties)
   2. Tube replacement: first planned tube change by ENT surgeon 5-7 days post surgery to allow tract maturation
   3. Prevent tube plugging: humidification of tracheostomy is essential to prevent crusting and tube blockage

4. Need for regular suctioning
5. Skin care (as risk of skin breakdown)
6. Appropriate nursing care on ward
7. Speech and language input if appropriate (feeding problems)
8. Provision of paper and pen to patient as they will be aphonic post tube insertion
9. Patient/caregiver education

d) It is a one way speaking valve, allowing airflow through the tracheostomy tube during inspiration only and during expiration the valve closes and air flows through the vocal cords

e)

1. Tracheostomy tube downsizing
2. Trial of capping (occlusive cap preventing airflow through tube) – never with cuff inflated!; must manage a full 24 hour period (usually over 2-3 days)
3. Original indication for tracheostomy must be resolved
4. Especially in paediatric tracheostomies a view from top (laryngoscopy) is necessary before decannulation to ensure no obstructive lesions (e.g. supra-stomal granulation)
5. Place airtight dressing to seal stoma after removal of tracheostomy with advice to apply pressure when talking/coughing

4.7 An intermittent facial swelling

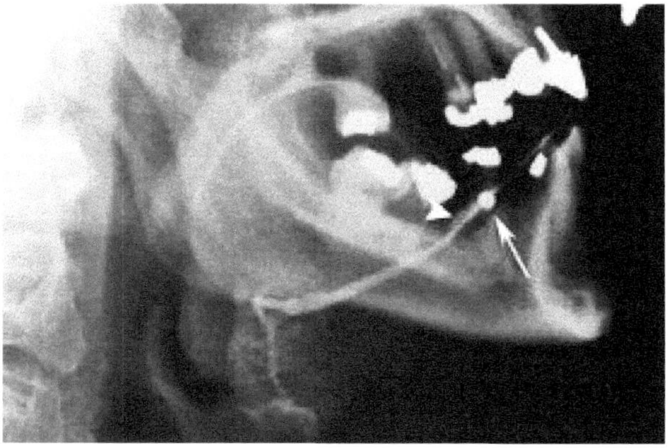

Questions

a) What investigation is being shown?

b) What is your diagnosis

c) Which gland is most commonly associated with this pathological process?

d) List 3 likely complications associated with this condition

e) For persistent cases, what are the most effective 2 treatments?

f) What investigations would you consider in a patient with recurrent symptoms, conjunctivitis sicca and xerostomia? List 2

Answers

a) Sialogram

b) Sialolithiasis

c) Submandibular gland (80%)

d)

   i. Fistula

   ii. Acute suppurative sialadenitis

   iii. Ductal stricture

e)

   i. Transoral sialodochoplasty or sialolithectomy

   ii. Submandibular gland excision

f) Most likely diagnosis would be Sjögrens. Would consider: Sublabial minor salivary gland biopsy (lymphocytic infiltrate) and autoantibodies (SS-A and SS-B)

4.8 Neck swelling in a child

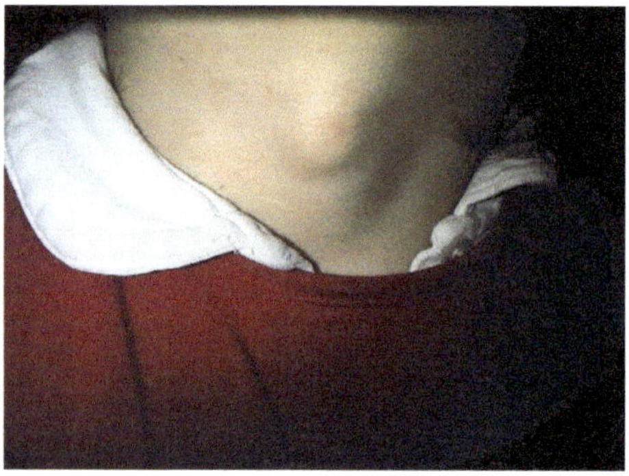

Questions

a) What is the most likely diagnosis?

b) Which is the single most useful investigation for this patient?

c) What would your differential include for a midline neck mass? List 3

d) What would your treatment options be for this patient?

e) What would surgery involve?

f) List 2 long-term complications of these masses?

Answers

a) Thyroglossal duct cyst

b) USS to confirm the presence of thyroid gland

c) Dermoid, sebaceous cyst, midline branchial cleft cyst, lymph node

d)

   i. Conservative

   ii. Surgical

e) Sistrunk procedure (excision of cyst, tract, including cuff of tongue base and midportion of hyoid bone)

f) Rarely malignant potential and secondary infections

4.9 An asymmetrical face

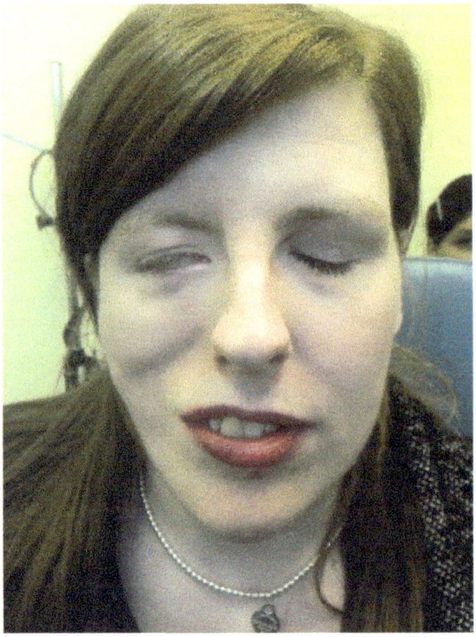

Questions

a) What is shown in the picture above

b) List 10 possible differentials

c) How is this condition graded?

d) Based on this grading system, what grade would represent normal function?

e) Based on this grading system, what grade would represent total paralysis?

f) What is critical when managing such patients?

Answers

a) A right-sided lower motor neurone facial nerve palsy.

b) Head trauma/temporal bone fracture, idiopathic (Bell's palsy), Ramsey-Hunt syndrome, otitis media, malignant otitis externa, cholesteatoma, post surgical (ear/parotid), parotid tumour, acoustic neuroma, diabetes mellitus

c) House-Brackman grading system

d) HB I

e) HB VI

f) Eye protection (artificial tears, ocular ointment and eye patch at night)

4.10 A wasted tongue

A 70-year old lady is seen in head and neck clinic for routine follow-up with an abnormal tongue.

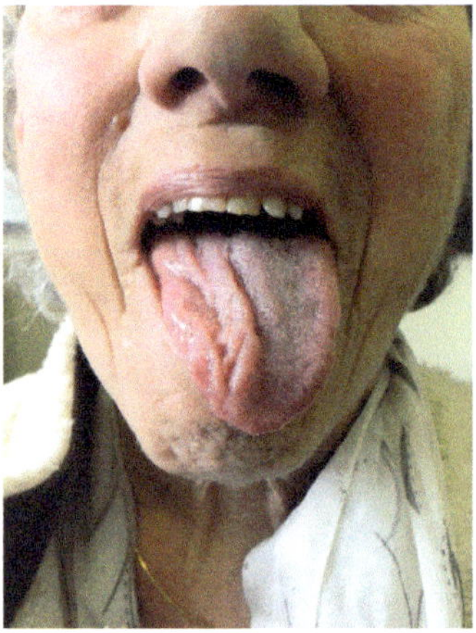

Questions

a) Describe the picture

b) What other signs might the patient have? List 2

c) What symptoms might this patient complain of? List 3

d) Which nerve is likely to have been injured

e) Where in the skull base does this nerve exit?

f) What operation might have injured it?

g) How is this nerve located intraoperatively?

Answers

a) Right sided hemitongue atrophy – smooth due to lack of papillae and loss of muscle bulk

b) May have scars of previous surgery, neck lump, worn dentition on contralateral side (eating on side away from the lesion)

c) Dysarthria, dysphagia, oral ulcers, worn dentition (from chewing on one side of mouth)

d) Right Hypoglossal nerve (CN XII)

e) Hypoglossal canal

f) Right submandibular gland excision

g) It is deep to the posterior belly of digastric

4.11 An angry looking neck lesion

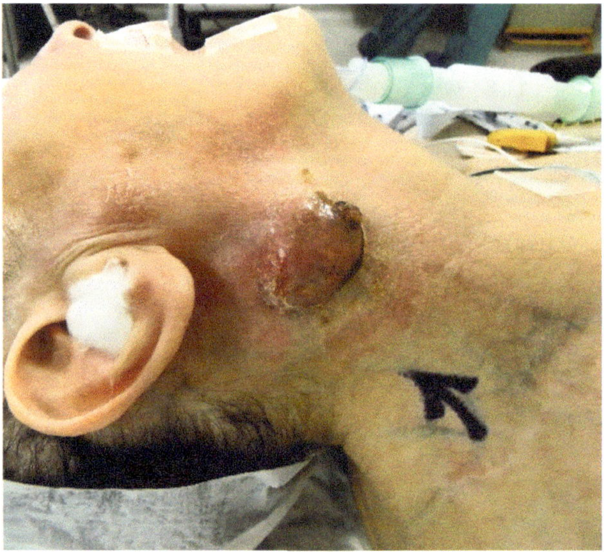

Questions

a) Describe the picture

b) What is the differential diagnosis?

c) What features of this lesion would lead you to suspect malignancy? List 5

d) What steps would you take in managing this patient?

Answers

a)

i. Anaesthetised marked patient with fungating lesion in the right tail of parotid region/level 2 neck

ii. Further skin changes in right pre-auricular region

b)

i. Primary cutaneous malignancy (eg SCC)

ii. Fungating tumour – eg lymph node or parotid

c) Pain, rapid growth, adherence to local structures, nerve involvement, neck nodes palpable

d) Ultrasound guided FNAC; MRI neck and CT chest to stage the disease; It is imperative to discuss the patient at a head and neck MDT

4.12 A furry tongue

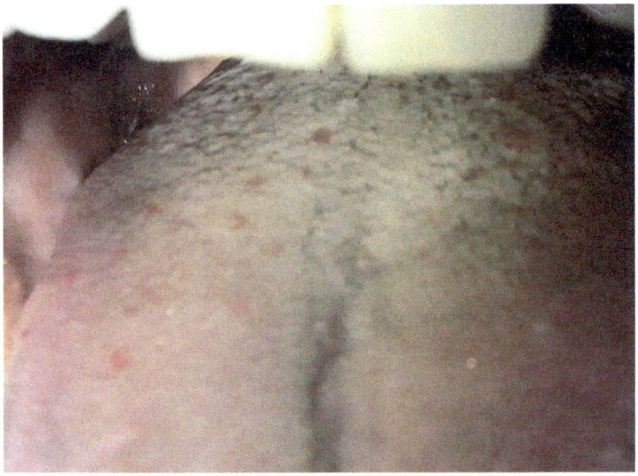

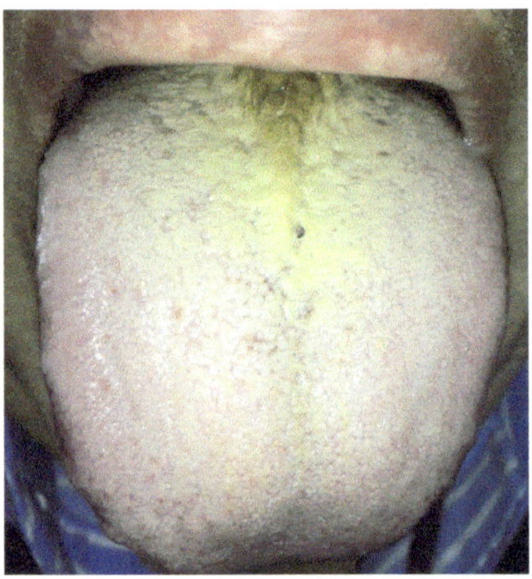

Questions

a) What types of papillae are found on the tongue?

b) What is the likely diagnosis in picture B?

c) What is the underlying process?

d) What is the aetiology?

e) What are the treatment options? List 6

Answers

a) There are 4 different types of papillae present on the tongue: fungiform, filiform, foliate and circumvallate

b) Clinical photograph of the dorsal surface of the tongue consistent with the diagnosis of a black hairy tongue

c) It is a condition of defective desquamation, hypertrophy and elongation of the filiform papillae which are present throughout the surface of the tongue

d) May be due to poor oral hygiene, low roughage diet, antibiotic usage or post-Radiotherapy. It is more common in males, especially those who smoke and drink lots of tea and coffee. Also increased incidence in HIV, IV drug usage. Higher incidence in incarcerated population.

e) (i) Lifestyle modification: Decreased caffeine intake, increased roughage in diet, improved oral hygiene, smoking cessation; (ii) Conservative: Tongue scraping, brushing; (iii) Surgery: Electrodessication, CO_2 laser, scissors

4.13 A fluid filled neck lump

A GP has referred a 30-year-old man with a left neck mass, which appeared following a viral upper respiratory tract infection.

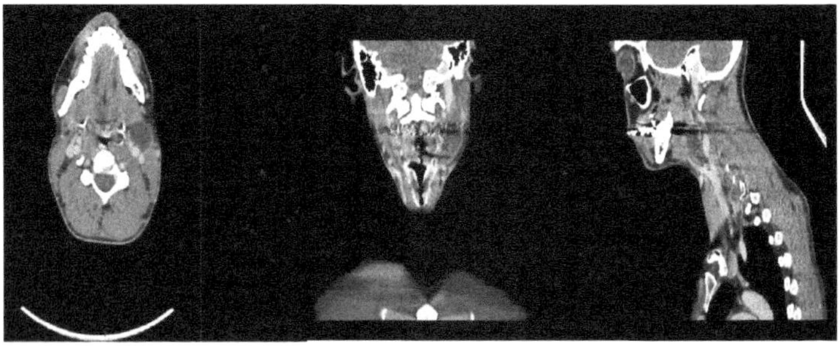

Questions

a) How would you approach this patient?

b) List two differential diagnoses other than branchial cyst

c) How would you investigate this patient. List 2

d) What is the typical description of fluid drained from a branchial cyst?

e) What is the pathogenesis of branchial cyst?

f) Assuming this is a branchial cyst, how would you manage this? List 2 options

Answers

a) History: Timing, infections, associated symptoms including airway compromise, dysphagia/odynophagia, weight loss, hoarseness, otalgia, smoking, alcohol

Examination: neck palpation, intra-oral examination, flexible nasendoscopy

b) Lymphadenopathy (reactive/infective)

   Neoplasm (primary or metastatic)

c) USS +/- FNA

   CT/MRI neck

d) Straw/cream-coloured, cloudy, low cellularity

e) Theories include branchial cleft remnant or trapped embryonic cells within a lymph node.

f) Surgical excision

   Watchful waiting – whilst it is not entirely unreasonable, the patient should be counselled that the cyst may persist or acutely enlarge following another infection causing potential airway compromise

4.14 Facial pain

Questions

A 50-year-old woman presents with a history of facial pain.

a) List 4 causes of facial pain

b) List 4 types of headache that may cause facial pain

c) If this facial pain was associated with a rash and facial weakness what would the causative organism likely to be?

d) What is the anatomical focus of this infection

e) What is the eponymous name given to this syndrome

f) Give 5 other features make up this syndrome. List 5

g) How would you treat this? List 3 options

Answers

a) Neurological, rhinological, otological, dental or TMJ-related, vascular, ophthamological

b) Tension headache, cluster headache, migraine, trigeminal neuralgia

c) Herpes zoster

d) Geniculate ganglion of facial nerve

e) Ramsay-Hunt syndrome

f) Hearing loss, vertigo, tinnitus, otalgia, taste disturbance

g) Analgesia, anti-virals, short course of high dose oral steroid if within 48h of presentation

4.15 Parapharyngeal mass

This 21 year old is seen in clinic with a 2-year history of gradually enlarging neck lump. It is found to be originating from the parapharyngeal space.

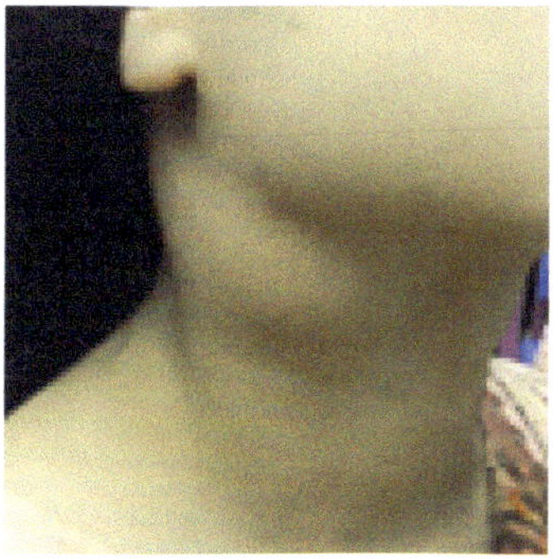

Questions

a) What are the boundaries of the parapharyngeal space

b) How are tumours of the parapharyngeal space classified?

c) What are the potential differential diagnoses?

d) How would this patient be managed? List 10 things

e) What are the surgical approaches to the parapharyngeal space?

f) What is the Lyre sign?

Answers

a) An inverted conical potential space with base at base of skull and apex at hyoid bone. Bounded by pharynx, parotid, mandible and pterygoid muscles:

b) The classification is anatomical and is based on the two compartments that are divided by the styloid process.

    i. Pre-styloid

    ii. Post-styloid

c) Pre-styloid: salivary gland tumours (benign and malignant)

   Post-styloid: schwannoma, paraganglioma, neurofibroma

d) History: duration, mass-effect, focal neurology, symptoms of excess catecholamines, family history

   Examination: inspect mass, palpation, pulsation, bruit, inspect oral cavity for medialisation of tonsils

   Investigations: CT scan of neck to assess mass, then proceed for FNAC if it is not vascular in origin; MRI may be able to give a radiological diagnosis but may not be able to show skull-base erosion; Proceed to surgical excision if required following discussion at appropriate MDT. If paraganglioma suspected will need endocrine review +/- genetics referral

e) Trans-cervical and trans-parotid

f) Splaying of the internal and external carotid, usually due to a carotid body tumour

4.16 Neck swelling in a child

This child is referred with a history of neck swelling since birth. The mass is smooth, compressible and transilluminates.

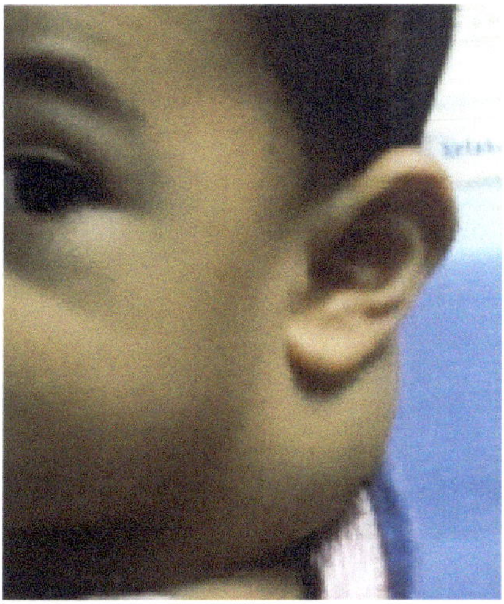

Questions

a) What is the most likely diagnosis?

b) What is the differential diagnosis? List 6

c) What complications might the mass present with? List 3

d) What imaging modality would be most suitable to get the diagnosis?

e) Suggest three management options

f) Name a staging system for this condition

g) Name two sclerosants

Answers

a) Cystic hygroma

b) Cervical cystic hygroma, haemangioma, teratoma, simple cyst, branchial cyst, cervical lymphadenopathy secondary to e.g. atypical mycobacteria

c) Infection, bleeding, airway obstruction

d) MRI

e) Watch and wait (5% resolve spontaneously), surgical excision, intralesional sclerotherapy

f)

   i. De Seres Classification (STAGE – LOCATION)

      1. Unilateral infrahyoid

      2. Unilateral suprahyoid

      3. Unilateral, supra and infrahyoid

      4. Bilateral suprahyoid

      5. Bilateral supra and infrahyoid

   ii. Giguere Classification

      1. Macrocystic – cystic spaces at least 2cm or more

      2. Microcystic – cystic spaces less than 2cm

      3. Mixed

g) Picibanil, Doxycycline – evoke an inflammatory response, causing fibrosis and obliteration of cell spaces

4.17 Facial sweating

You see this patient in clinic who has had a parotidectomy. He complains of facial sweating on the same side as the surgery.

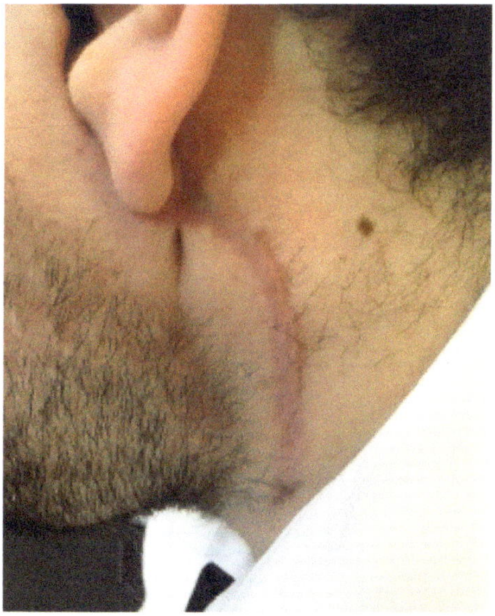

Questions

a. What is the name of this incision and name an alternative incision that can be used for parotidectomy?

b. What is the name of the condition described by the patient?

c. Name 2 options for management of this condition

d. Damage to which nerve causes a numb ear lobule?

e. Name 2 differential diagnoses of a parotid enlargement?

Answers

a. Blair incision (or modified Blair incision) and rhytidectomy or face lift incision

b. Frey's syndrome

c. Aluminium based deodorant, topical glycopyrrolate, botulinum toxin injection, glossopharyngeal neuronectomy

d. Great auricular nerve

e. Parotitis, pleomorphic adenoma, granulomatous disease

4.18 An intra-oral lesion above the tongue

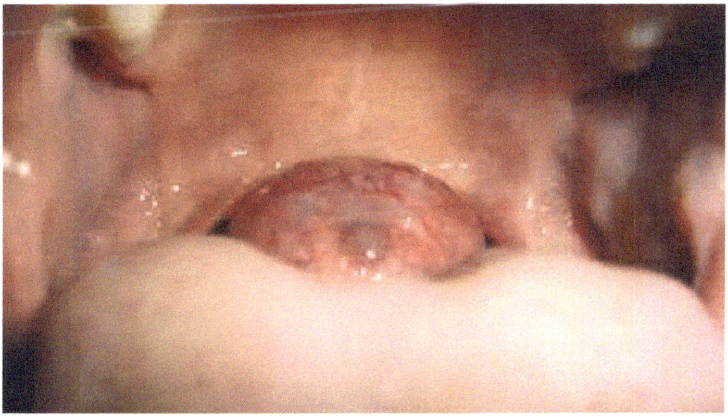

Questions

a) What is the differential diagnosis? List 5

b) What investigation would help to determine the diagnosis?

c) What symptoms may the patient present with? List 2

d) What are the management options?

e) List the most common sites of ectopic thyroid. List 3

Answers

a) Lingual thyroid, thyroglossal duct cyst, midline branchial cleft cyst, lymphangioma, dermoid cyst, minor salivary gland tumour, tongue base tumour

b) Technetium Tc-99m sodium thyroid scan

c) Most ectopic tissue is asymptomatic but may increase in size and become symptomatic during puberty and pregnancy. It is four times more common in females.

They may bleed, and malignant transformation has been reported

d) Trans-oral resection or trans-cervical pharyngostomy and a covering tracheostomy. Post-operative T4 replacement may be given to suppress ectopic thyroid tissue recurrence

e) Lingual, sublingual, pre-tracheal, mediastinal

4.19 An intra-oral lesion below the tongue

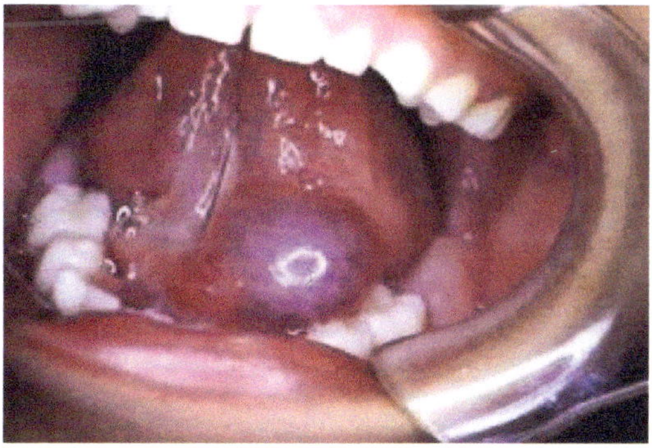

a) What is the differential? List 4

b) What tests may be performed to confirm the diagnosis?

c) How may the condition be managed?

d) What can complicate the removal of such a lesion?

e) Can this be a congenital lesion?

Answers

a) Extravasation mucocoele (ranula), lymphangioma, dermoid cyst, supra-hyoid thyroglossal duct cyst, ectopic thyroid

b) Aspiration of the pseudocyst, MRI

c) Surgical excision, including the sublingual gland

d) The cyst may extend through the floor of the mouth into the neck (plunging ranula)

e) Congenital ranula may occur, probably as a result of thumb sucking *in utero* which may damage any part of the sublingual gland.

4.20 Anterior neck swelling

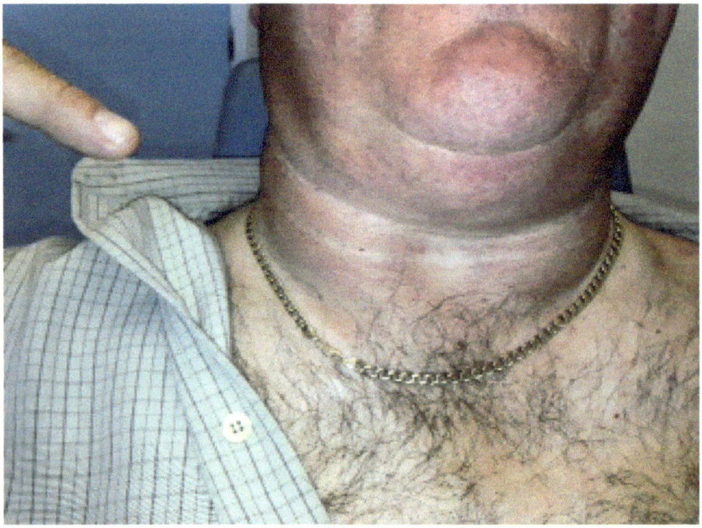

Questions

a) What is the abnormality present in the photograph?

b) List 5 possible causes for this condition

c) Give 5 symptoms which may be present

d) List 3 indications for surgery

e) What are five possible complications of surgical treatment?

Answers

a) Goitre

b) Multinodular goitre; Graves' disease; Infective thyroiditis; granulomatous disease such as sarcoidosis; Iodine deficiency; Thyroid cancer.

c) Dyspnoea, dysphagia, Graves' related eye disorder; tremor-associated hypo, Dysphonia; Symptoms of hyperthyroidism

d) Neck lump greater than 4cm, pressure symptoms leading to dyspnoea or dysphagia, weak voice, or suspicion of malignancy

e) Bleeding, infection, hypocalcaemia, recurrent laryngeal nerve palsy, pneumothorax

CHAPTER 5

Imaging in Head and Neck

5.1 MRI Parapharyngeal lesion

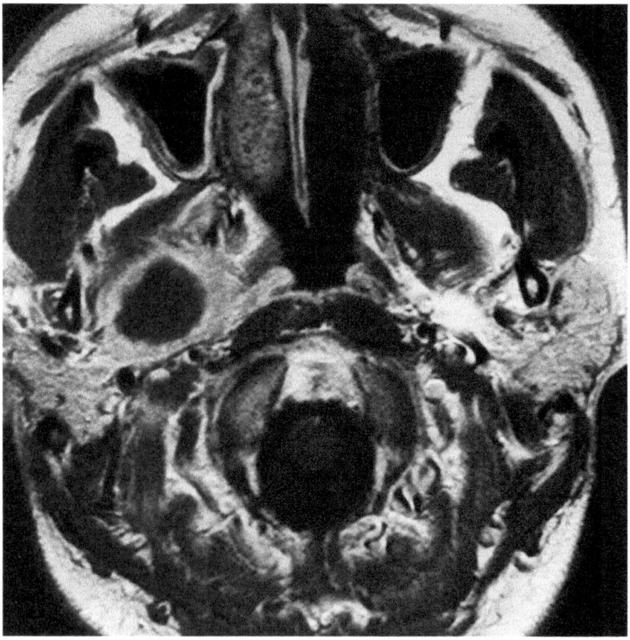

Questions

a) What type of scan is shown above?

b) Which part of the neck is this image showing?

c) What abnormality is seen

d) Give 2 possible diagnoses

Answers

a) Axial MRI T1-weighted with contrast

b) Suprahyoid neck through the parapharyngeal space

c) A ring enhancing lesion with central low signal in the right parapharyngeal space

d) Parapharyngeal abscess or branchial cyst

5.2 MRI bilateral schwannomas

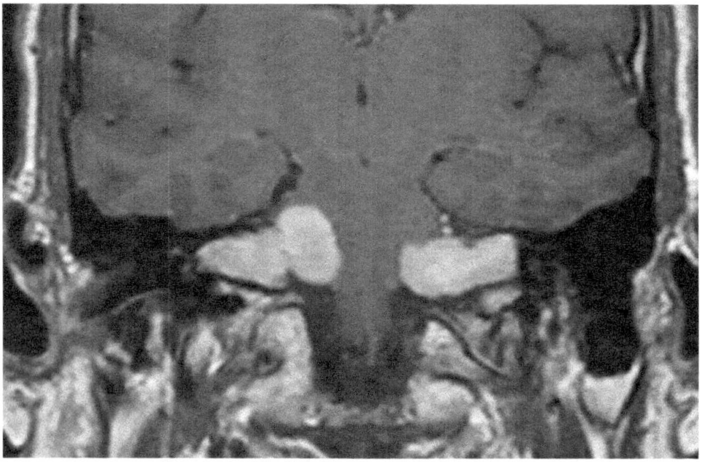

Questions

a) What plane is this scan?

b) What is this investigation?

c) Describe the abnormality shown

d) What is the most likely name of the lesions shown?

e) Which conditions might this patient be suffering from?

f) How would you rehabilitate the hearing loss if this patient had surgery to remove the lesions?

Answers

a) Coronal

b) MRI T1 weighted with contrast

c) Bilateral lesions in the cerebellopontine angles

d) Acoustic neuromas or vestibular schwannomas

e) Neurofibromatosis type 2

f) Brainstem implants

5.3 CT unilateral sinus lesion

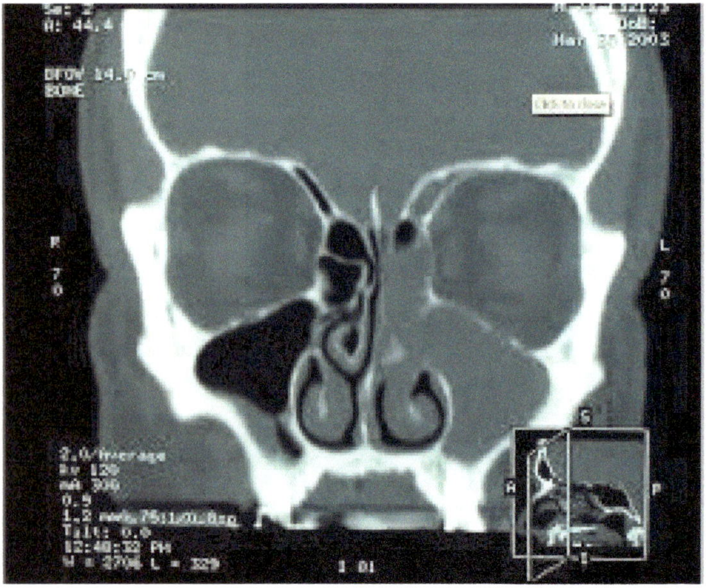

Questions

a) What is this view?

b) What is this investigation?

c) Describe the abnormality shown

d) Damage to which artery may cause increased intra-ocular pressure?

e) List 6 important structures that can be damaged during FESS surgery?

Answers

a) Coronal view

b) Computerised tomography (CT) scan of the sinuses

c) There is opacification of the left maxillary and ethmoid sinuses. There is a concha bullosa on the right side and mild maxillary mucosal thickening.

d) Anterior ethmoidal artery (branch of the internal carotid artery)

e) Optic nerve, medial rectus muscle, skull base, nasolacrimal duct, infra-orbital nerve

5.4 CT scan of temporal bone

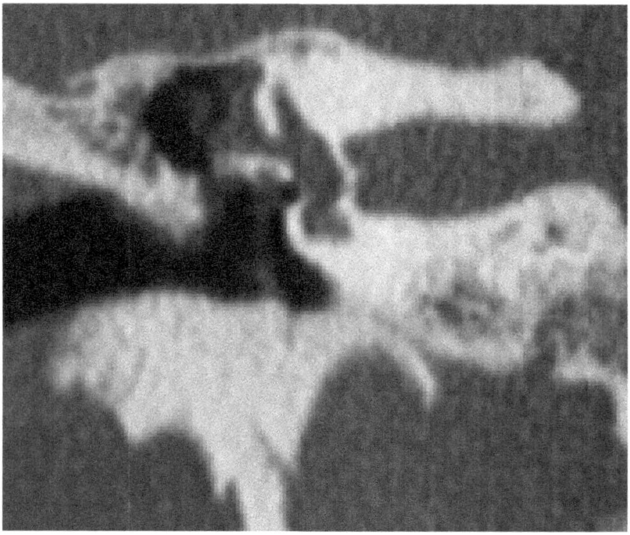

Questions

a) What plane is this scan?

b) What abnormality is seen

c) What is the most likely cause for the abnormality?

d) What sign may be elicited in the clinic

e) How is the condition treated

Answers

a) Coronal CT of temporal bone

b) Lateral semicircular fistula

c) Cholesteatoma

d) Positive fistula test

e) Tympanomastoid surgery with grafting of the fistula with temporalis fascia

5.5 A patient with smell disturbance

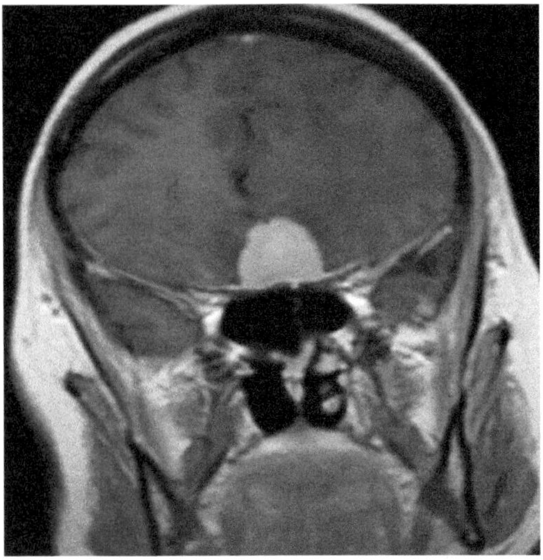

Questions

a) What type of scan is shown above?

b) Describe the abnormality

c) What is the most likely diagnosis?

d) List 2 symptoms this patient may present with

Answers

a) Coronal MRI T1-weighted with contrast

b) A broad base lesion with bilateral dural tail above the sphenoid sinus

c) A olfactory groove meningioma

d) Anosmia and headache

5.6 CT inner ear deformity

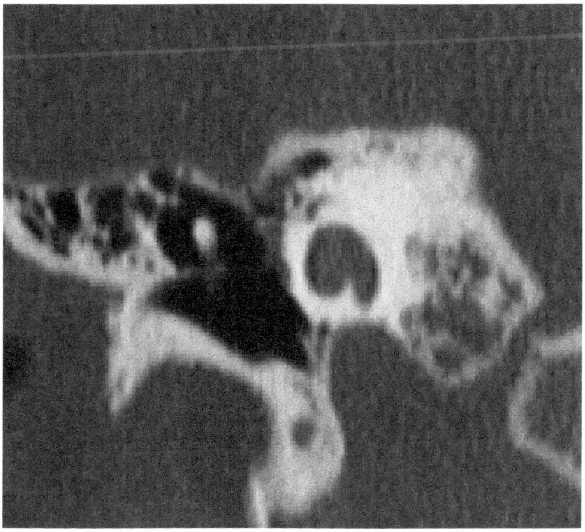

Questions

a) What is the anatomical plane of this image?

b) What is the abnormality shown in this image?

c) What symptom may this patient experience?

d) How might this be treated?

e) What association are there with this condition?

Answers

a) Coronal CT of temporal bone

b) Mondini malformation of cochlea

c) Sensorineural deafness

d) Cochlear implant

e) Rubella and thalidomide

5.7 CT Scan of the temporal bone

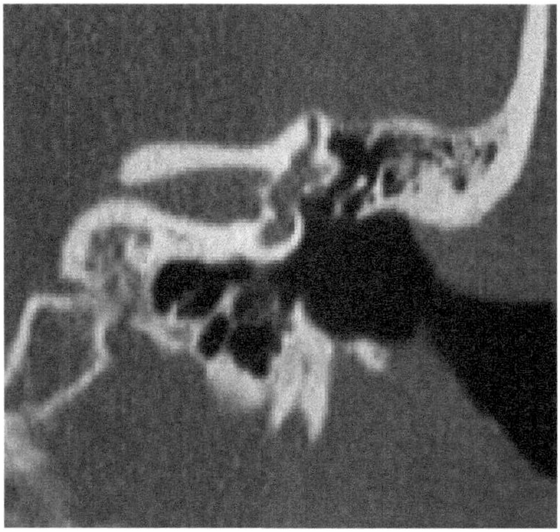

Questions

a) What type of imaging is shown above?

b) What is the main finding of the scan?

c) List 5 symptoms this patient might present with

d) In this condition, what type of hearing loss is most likely to be present?

e) How would you manage this patient? List 6 things

f) What are the treatment options?

Answers

a) A coronal CT scan of the left temporal bone

b) Superior semicircular canal dehiscence

c) Tullio phenomenon (vertigo or dizziness induced by loud sound); autophony (person's own speech or self generated noises such as chewing perceived as unusually loud); dizziness/vertigo; hyperacusis; hearing loss; aural fullness; pulsatile tinnitus, headache

d) Conductive hearing loss due to inner ear third mobile window

e) History

Examination (including full ENT/head and neck exam & cranial nerves)

Imaging (HRCT of temporal bone if not already done)

Audiological assessment (e.g. PTA, tympanogram, and acoustic reflexes)

f) **Conservative** (e.g. avoidance of loud sounds/exacerbating trigger; reassurance)

Surgical (e.g. resurfacing defect or plugging superior canal)

5.8 CT microtia

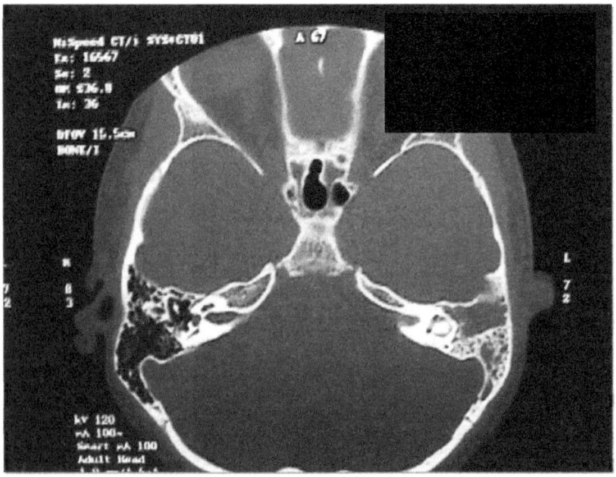

Questions

a) What type of scan is this?

b) Name 2 abnormalities present.

c) What type of hearing loss is likely to be present?

d) Assuming the inner ear is normal, what is the maximum conductive hearing loss this patient may have?

e) What type of hearing aid is suitable for this patient?

f) List 4 syndromes/sequences associated with this type of scan

Answers

a) Axial CT scan of the temporal bone (bony window)

b) Unilateral microtia and sclerotic mastoid on the left side

c) Conductive hearing loss due to absence of ear canal and perhaps ossicular dysfunction

d) 60dB

e) Bone conduction hearing aid e.g. BAHA

f) Goldenhaar's, Treacher-Collins, Pierre-Robin sequence, CHARGE

5.9 X-ray neck prevertebral soft tissue swelling

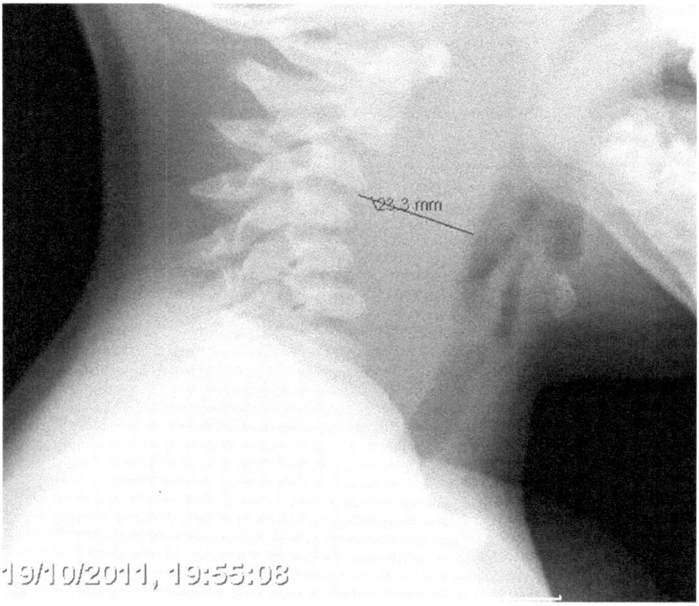

Questions

a) List 4 causes for the swelling of the prevertebral soft tissue in the x-ray above

b) What is the normal thickness of the prevertebral soft tissue

c) Assuming this is an infective process, list 4 possible complications

d) Which neck muscle is important to identify whilst during cervical draining of a parapharyngeal space lesion?

Answers

a) Parapharyngeal abscess, retropharyngeal abscess, foreign body and severe URTI

b) 7mm in front of C1-C4 and 1.7mm in front of C5-C8

c) Mediastinitis, mediastinal abscess, purulent pericarditis, bronchial erosion, aspiration pneumonia

d) Digastric (posterior belly)

5.10 MRI Sinonasal tumour

A 55-year old furniture maker has been referred to you with a 6 months history of progressive left-sided nasal obstruction. More recently, he has been suffering with intermittent nasal discharge, scabbing and epistaxis. Here are images pertaining to the patient.

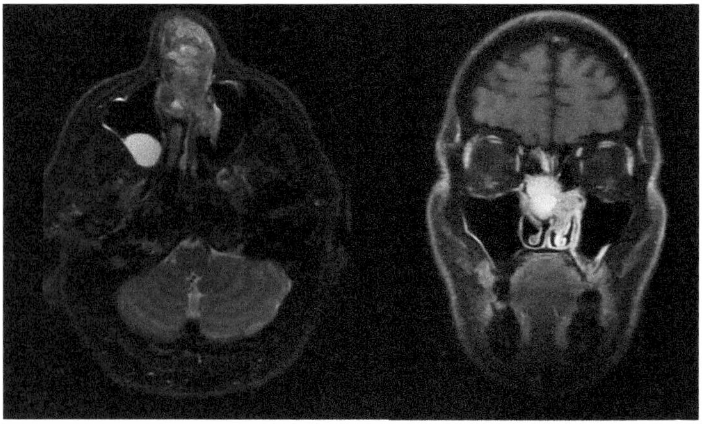

Questions

a) What type of scan is shown above?

b) Please describe the images above

c) Would you biopsy this in clinic?

d) What is the differential diagnosis? List 5

e) What is the most likely diagnosis?

Answers

a) T1 weighted MRI with contrast

b) Axial MRI scan demonstrating a left sided lesion occluding the entire nasal cavity with deviation of the septum to the right. Coronal MRI scan more posteriorly showing that the mass does not appear to involve the skull base, posterior ethmoids and orbit

c) No – risk of bleed / CSF leak if intracranial extension. Biopsy under GA in a controlled environment

d) Benign: Inverting papilloma, antrochoanal polyp, meningoencephalocoele

   Malignant: Adenocarcinoma, squamous cell carcinoma, esthesioblastoma

e) Adenocarcinoma (because he is a carpenter and most likely works with hard wood)

CHAPTER 6

Manned Stations

6. 1 A patient with a feeling of something in the throat

Brief	A 35-year-old female lawyer presents with a history of a lump in the throat. Take a history and then Answer the examiner's questions.

Gel hands, introduce yourself and ask permission to talk

Introduction, brief demographics:

How old is the patient and what is their employment (will often be relevant)

Presenting complaint:

What exactly is the problem in the patient's own words?

History of the presenting complaint:

Temporal factors: When did it start, How long has it been there, is it constant / intermittent.

Associated factors: Any other associated symptoms, is it worse with eating or does it go? Is it only present when you swallow your saliva rather than when you are eating and drinking?

Red flags: Dysphagia, odynophagia, otalgia, regurgitation of foods, solids vs liquids, weight-loss, voice change, neck lumps

Systemic enquiry:

Constitutional symptoms: Weight loss, fevers, night sweats, fatigue, itching.

Past medical history:

Gastro-oesophageal reflux disease, mental health problems, ingestion of caustic substances.

Social History:

Does the patient smoke or drink alcohol or use other illicit drugs?

Ask about current stresses – what is the patient worried about? If you have built a rapport the patient will share their ideas, concerns and expectations. The patient's main concern may be about cancer.

Drug history:

Has the patient used PPI's in the past, or are they on any other medications.

Examiner's Question:

How would you manage this patient?

Model answer

This patient most likely has Globus Pharyngeus. In the absence of red flag symptoms, and with normal examination findings (Clinical and Flexible nasendoscopy), this patient, who is under 40 and does not smoke or drink, can be reassured that the likelihood of this being anything sinister is unlikely and any further investigation is unnecessary.

If there were any red-flag features, then the patient

should be given a full head and neck examination, barium swallow or CT scan plus a possible panendoscopy and biopsy.

6.2 Explaining the diagnosis of cholesteatoma to the mother of a patient

Brief	This 10 year old boy has been given a diagnosis of cholesteatoma. His mother is here in clinic today – please explain the diagnosis and Answer the questions she has.

Gel hands, introduce yourself and ask permission to talk

Information gathering:

Check her understanding and gauge her level of anxiety.

'I have been told that your son has been diagnosed with cholesteatoma. I know this is perhaps worrying for you – what do you understand so far and can I help to explain the condition?'

Information giving:

Explain that cholesteatoma is a ball of skin cells that is growing in the middle ear - use a diagram to show this.

'The ear is divided into the outer ear, middle ear and inner ear. You son has skin cells growing here that are in the wrong place'.

'How did this happen?'

'We are not quite sure why this happens however there are a few theories. People are either born with them or develop them later in life. It is sometimes related to a pocket in the ear drum because of a blocked Eustachian tube (refer to diagram) or following damage to the eardrum from infections or surgery.'

'What needs to be done?'

'The risk of leaving this untreated is that complications can develop, some of which can be life threatening. Although the yearly risk is low, over a lifetime this can become high. We therefore recommend surgery.'

6.3 Examination of the balance system

Brief	Please examine this patient's balance system – you DO NOT need to take a history

Gel hands, introduce yourself and ask permission to talk

'Hello, my name is Doctor X, I've been asked to examine your balance system today – is that OK. Firstly are you in any pain?

Cerebellum

Dysdiadochokinesis

Ataxia

Nystagmus

Intention tremor

Slurred speech (dysarthria)

Hypotonia

Eye Movements

Nystagmus

Otoscopy

Check for ear pathology

Cranial nerve examination

Specifically vestibulocochlear nerve (CN VIII) and Facial nerve (CN VII)

Proprioception

Joint position sense

Balance

Romberg's & Unterberger's tests, Head Thrust and Dix-Hallpike test

6.4 Giving bad news – a patient with a T1aN0M0 laryngeal cancer

Brief	This patient has had previous microlaryngoscopy with biopsy (MLB), histology is now back showing T1aN0M0 laryngeal cancer – please give this information to the patient and answer any questions they may have.

Gel hands, introduce yourself and ask permission to talk:

'Hello Mr Jones, my name is Dr X, one of the ENT doctors working in clinic today.

Information gathering:

'Have you brought anyone with you today? – Would you like someone to be here?'

'What do you understand about the tests we have done so far?'

Information giving:

A warning shot:

'I'm afraid I have bad news' / 'I'm afraid the results are not what we hoped for'

Give information slowly and without jargon:

'The growth in your voice-box is an early cancer. As we have found this early, it has not had time to spread. We are therefore confident that with the right treatment we will be able to remove it entirely'.

Answer questions openly and honestly:

'I'm afraid I don't know the answer to that as it is carried out by doctors from another specialty – I can check with a colleague and let you know shortly'.

Closure and summary:

Bring the discussion to a close by asking the patient if there is anything else, offer them a leaflet or support contact. Summarise the consultation and offer them an appointment in the future should they wish to discuss anything further.

6.5 Head and Neck examination

Brief	Examine this patient's neck

Gel hands, introduce yourself and ask permission to examine the patient

Adequately position and expose the patient

The patient should be sitting with collar loosened to show clavicles, check the patient is comfortable.

Inspection

Look at the patient are there any signs of flushing, an obvious neck / facial mass or facies suggesting hypo/hyperthyroidism? Are there any features of malignancy including cachexia?

Ask the patient to take a mouthful of water and swallow whilst observing for a mass.

Palpation

Ask the patient to take a mouthful of water and swallow again – this time feeling for a mass moving with the swallow.

Percussion

Percuss over the neck mass in the midline and down the sternum for the characteristic dullness of retrosternal mass such as a goitre.

Auscultation

Listen over the neck for a bruit

Offer to perform oral examination and FNE

6.6 Flexible nasendoscopy

Brief	Perform FNE on this patient and answer the examiner's questions

Gel hands, introduce yourself and ask permission to examine the patient

Offer to perform brief anterior rhinoscopy on the patient to assess for gross obstruction

Give the patient a choice of nostril to pass the 'scope and the option of local anaesthetic – explain not to drink hot fluids for two hours after the procedure

Pick up the nasendoscope and lubricate tip as well as using demisting pad for the tip

Focus 'scope on text of the demisting pad

Introduce the 'scope tip, warning the patient beforehand, use little finger of hand holding tip to steady against the patients nose tip

Offer to halt the procedure if patient is concerned/in pain

Offer reassurance throughout the examination, patient is to sit up and breathe normally through the mouth

Comment on the structures visible as you pass – Turbinates, nasal septum, PNS, Eustachian tube openings, fossae of Rosenmüller, tonsils, posterior pharyngeal wall, tongue base, vallecula, larynx including position and movement of cords (mucosal wave of cord on phonation can only be commented upon under a stroboscope)

Ask the patient to protrude tongue and perform Valsalva manoeuvre (to visualise the Vallecula and Piriform fossae respectively)

Advise the patient that the 'scope is being withdrawn. Offer a tissue and a glass of water, apologise for any discomfort caused

Examiner's question: *Can you please draw this patient's larynx? (Normal anatomy)*

6.7 Examination of ears and facial nerve

Brief	Examine the ears and facial nerve of this patient.

Ears

Gel hands, introduce yourself and ask permission to examine the patient

Ask if they have any pain

Examine the patient's external ears using light of the otoscope

Comment on symmetry, size, presence of hearing aid

Look in front of the ear for pre-auricular pits/sinuses and any subtle scar from 'facelift' or endaural incision

Look behind the ear, pulling pinna forward to look for mastoid scars, swelling – ask about tenderness before palpating

Check the scalp for evidence of a BAHA

Look into the ear with otoscope

Comment on canal and debris

Comment on the ear drum (MIPC)

Malleus

Is the drum **Intact**

Pars tensa and flaccida

What is the **position** of the drum?

Comment on the **colour** of the drum

Perform fistula test and Rinne and Weber's tests, offer

free field tests

Offer FNE to inspect PNS and Eustachian tube orifices

Facial nerve

Systematic examination of the temporal, zygomatic, buccal, marginal mandibular and cervical branches of CN VII

Inspect the patients face for symmetry

Temporal – ask patient to raise eyebrows, comment on symmetry of frontalis elevation

If asymmetry is there sparing of forehead? – if sparing it is UMN lesion (remember bicortical representation of the forehead facial motor nucleus)

Zygomatic – Scrunch up eyes – test against resistance

Buccal - Puff out cheeks – test against resistance

Mandibular - Show teeth

Remember facial nerve sensory branch – chorda tympani

Offer to test taste for anterior third of the tongue

Examiner's questions

This patient has a rash in the ear and dense facial nerve palsy with forehead involvement on the same side. What is the diagnosis? can you name the causative organism?

How do you grade the facial palsy and how will you manage this?

Model answer:

'This patient is likely to have the Ramsay-Hunt syndrome. This is caused by reactivation of latent herpes zoster infection in the geniculate ganglion of the facial nerve'.

'The facial palsy can be graded using the House-Brackman scale (this has been criticised for having poor inter-observer reproducibility), and treatment is primarily symptomatic, including eye protection and antivirals/steroids if the patient presents in the first 48 hours'.

6.8 Epistaxis history and Examination of nose

Brief	Take a history from this patient who suffers from epistaxis and then perform anterior rhinoscopy – answer the examiner's questions.

Gel hands, introduce yourself and ask permission to examine the patient

Presenting complaint

What has brought you to clinic today? / I understand you have come to clinic today with nosebleeds

History of the presenting complaint

Tell me what happens with your bleeds

Temporal questions

Onset (eg nose-blowing)

Duration

How long have you had these for?

Does anything make it better?

Does anything seem to make it worse?

Do you feel unwell with them or have any other associated symptoms? – e.g. bruising (haematological conditions)

Have you had a recent cold/flu, trauma to the nose e.g. nose picking

Past medical history

Do you have: high blood pressure, problems with the blood clotting or a history of bleeding from any other part of the body? (e.g. stomach/bowels)

Any previous nasal surgery?

Drug history

Do you take any medicines to thin the blood (Aspirin, clopidogrel, warfarin, factor Xa antagonsists)?

Do you use nasal steroid sprays?

Social history

Who lives with you? (important for discharge planning)

Do you take any illicit drugs through the nose?

Do you pick your nose?

Family history

Does anyone in the family get regular nosebleeds?

Does anyone have a history of hereditary haemorrhagic telangiectasia?

Check the patient's understanding and Ideas, concerns and expectations

'What were you hoping to find out in clinic today?'

'Are you satisfied that we have explored your concerns today?'

Anterior rhinoscopy

Explain the procedure to the patient – *'I need to examine your nose buy looking into the nostrils with this instrument – it should not be painful, please let me know if you want me to stop / sneeze etc.'*

Ask about pain or tenderness

Appearance

Comment on the external nose, looking from the front, sides and top

Look carefully for scars

Anatomy

Comment on abnormal anatomy eg dorsal hump, tip ptosis or deviation of nasion

Function

Use Lack's speculum to test for patency

Look for alar collapse

Offer to perform validated smell tests (e.g. UPSIT)

Internally

Hold Thuddicum's speculum correctly and examine gently both nostrils with head-torch

Comment on turbinates and nasal septum

Reassure patient as you progress

Offer FNE to visualise PNS and posterior septum and well as Eustachian tube orifices

Thank the patient and offer them a tissue

Examiner's question

On examining the patient you notice a telangiectatic rash on the patients oral mucosa, he divulges that his father had nosebleeds and died of an intestinal haemorrhage – he isn't sure as they weren't close and he grew up with his mother.

What condition may this patient have? What is the mechanism of inheritance and the pathophysiology?

Model answer

'This patient may have hereditary haemorrhagic telangiectasia (HHT), or Osler-Weber-Rendu disease. This is an autosomal dominant condition.'

6.9 Explanation of unilateral SNHL to father of 2 year old. The father is interested in the 'bionic ear'

Brief	This two-year-old boy has been diagnosed with a unilateral dead ear. Explain the diagnosis to his father and then answer any questions he may have.

Introduce yourself by name and role, ask permission to speak with the patient

Check the person's relationship to the patient

Check their understanding

> *'Your son has been referred to clinic for his hearing, he had some tests and I understand that you would like to discuss the results of these'.*

Ask if there is anyone else who may want to be in the consultation

Fire a warning shot

> *'I have some news that may be upsetting about your son's hearing' – allow patient time to react*

> *'Would you like me to continue?'*

Give explanation

> *'The hearing tests show that he has no hearing on the left hand side, here is a diagram showing the ear – it can be divided into, outer, middle and inner. It is likely that your son has a problem with the inner ear which is comprised of the cochlear and auditory nerve.'*

What caused this? Why wasn't it picked up sooner?

> *'The reasons behind this are not always clear; sometimes there is an association with other conditions.*

In this case however there is no other association and it is not helpful to do other tests. It was not picked up sooner as the tests that we perform at birth are not 100% sensitive and also he has compensated very well with his good ear.'

What can be done to improve this?

'He may benefit from a bone anchored hearing aid on a headband which will help with sound localisation, it is also important to protect the 'good' ear as this will be relied upon in the future'.

6.10 Explanation of indication for tonsillectomy

Brief	This 11-year-old child has been admitted with an episode of tonsillitis, the 3rd this year, having had three episodes in each of the last 3 years. Explain to the patient's family the diagnosis and the management options. The parents are very keen to proceed to tonsillectomy – is this an option, if not, why?

Introduce yourself by name and role; ask permission to speak with the patient

Check the parents' understanding of why a tonsillectomy is performed

> *'A tonsillectomy is performed in people who get recurrent severe infections of the tonsils'.*

It is helpful to know the current SIGN guidelines regarding tonsillectomy:

- sore throats are due to acute tonsillitis
- the episodes of sore throat are disabling and prevent normal functioning
- seven or more well documented, clinically significant, adequately treated sore

  throats in the preceding year or
- five or more such episodes in each of the preceding two years or
- three or more such episodes in each of the preceding three years.

Explain the anatomy and briefly explain how a tonsillectomy is performed

> *'The tonsils are found in the back of the throat on both sides (a diagram may help). Generally, viral infections cause them to grow large and become painful. They may then become infected with bacteria, which is why your GP may offer you antibiotics'.*

Explain the risks of tonsillectomy and the aftercare needed

> *'The main risks of tonsillectomy are bleeding, infection, pain and very rarely damage to teeth. Bleeding can occur early or later, the latter is usually due to infection. Rarely bleeding is severe and some patients will need a further operation to deal with this. It is important to take adequate pain relief and to eat a normal diet as a soon as possible – this is thought to reduce the risk of bleeding.'*

6.11 Explanation of indications for myringoplasty

Brief	This 13-year-old boy has been referred to clinic with a persistently discharging ear resulting from a perforated drum that has not healed – counsel the parents about the indications for a myringoplasty.

Introduce yourself by name and role; ask permission to speak with the patient

Check the person's relationship to the patient

Check their understanding

> *'I understand your son has a had trouble with a discharging ear and that you are here to discuss the treatment options for this'*

Offer an explanation of the procedure

> *'Sometimes a hole in the ear drum does not heal and as a result the middle ear produces fluid that discharges out of the ear canal. This can be troublesome for the patient as well as causing embarrassment socially. It can also prevent you from carrying out activities such as swimming.'*
>
> *'This operation is performed not to improve hearing, but to cover the eardrum in order to prevent discharge and allow activities such as swimming'*
>
> *'A piece of tissue, called 'fascia' from behind the ear is used as a graft to plug the hole in the eardrum.'*
>
> *'There are several ways of performing this operation, all under a general anaesthetic. You may have a cut in the ear canal or hidden in the crease behind the ear.'*
>
> *'After the operation he will wake up with a head*

bandage, and some packing in the ear. The bandage will come off the next day and the dressing in the ear will be removed after a week in clinic.'

'As with all operations there are some potential complications, including bleeding, infection and failure of the graft. Some patients may have deterioration in hearing. Very rarely there is a total loss of hearing. Similarly there is very small risk of taste disturbance or vertigo. The latter should settle soon after surgery'

Offer the parents/patient an opportunity to express their ideas, concerns and expectations

The parents may have thought that the operation was intended to improve hearing , and place the discharge from the ear low down the list of concerns.

Answer any questions the patient might have

How long before he can go swimming / fly in a plane / need for post-operative drops etc.

6.12 Consent for parotidectomy for pleomorphic adenoma

Brief	Please take consent from this patient for the above operation.

Introduce yourself by name and role; ask permission to speak with the patient

Check the person's name – make sure it matches with any documentation

Check their understanding

> *'I understand that you are here today to discuss an operation to remove the gland in your cheek that produces saliva – the parotid gland.'*
>
> *'you have been found to have a growth in the saliva gland called a pleiomorphic adenoma. Although this is benign, there is a risk that it may become malignant if left alone for a long time (1% cumulative risk per annum after 10 years).'*

Explain the operation

> *'A parotidectomy is an operation to remove the gland through a cut on the side of the face, usually hidden in the skin crease.*
>
> *You will normally come into hospital the day before the operation. The operation usually lasts a few hours and afterwards you will wake up with a dressing on your face and a drain. You will need to stay in hospital until the drain has been taken out – usually 24h.'*

Explain the complications

> *'With any operation there is a risk of bleeding and infection. The parotid gland is closely related to the nerve*

that supplies the muscles in the face. If this is damaged, then the face may be paralysed on that side. Sometimes the nerve is bruised, in which case function will return, if the nerve is cut however then it is unlikely to recover'.

'A lot of care is taken however to protect this nerve and a special monitor is attached to the face to help prevent this complication'

'Another possible complication is caused by nerves growing from where the gland is, into the skin over it – this can lead to flushing/sweating of skin when you are eating. This can be managed and often improves over time.'

Offer that parents/patient an opportunity to express their ideas, concerns and expectations

The parents may have concerns regarding cosmesis, or be unaware of the risks of malignant transformation

Answer any questions the patient might have

'How long before I can wash my face / wear make-up / return to work' etc.

6.13 Consent for submandibular gland excision

Brief	Please take consent from this patient for the above operation.

Introduce yourself by name and role; ask permission to speak with the patient

Check the person's relationship to the patient

Check their understanding

'I understand that you are here today to discuss an operation to remove the gland under your jaw that produces saliva – the submandibular gland.'

'You have had issues with stones causing a blockage here and have been advised that an operation to remove it would give you relief from your symptoms.'

'removing the gland will have little effect on your saliva production as the other gland will be able to compensate.'

Explain the operation

'The purpose of the operation is to remove the submandibular gland through a cut in the skin crease under the jaw.'

'You will normally come into hospital the day of the operation. The operation usually lasts a few hours and afterwards you will wake up with a dressing on your face. You will usually be able to go home the same day.'

Explain the complications

'As with any operation there is a risk of bleeding and infection. The submandibular gland is closely related to

the nerve that supplies the tongue and the corner of the mouth. If this is damaged, then the tongue may be paralysed on that side, or the mouth droop on that side. Sometimes the nerve is bruised, in which case function will return, if the nerve is cut however then it is unlikely to recover'.

'A lot of care is taken to protect these nerves and complications like this are rare '

Offer that parents/patient an opportunity to express their ideas, concerns and expectations

The patient may have concerns re the cosmesis or have been unaware of the potential complications

Answer any questions the patient might have

'How long before I can wash my face / wear make-up / return to work' etc.

6.14 Counsel the parent of a child with suspected sleep-disordered breathing

Brief	This parent has just seen a program on TV regarding sleep disordered breathing and is concerned that her child may have obstructive sleep apnoea because she is a heavy snorer and a mouth breather. Counsel her regarding sleep-disordered breathing by first explaining what it is all about.

Introduce yourself by name and role; ask permission to speak with the patient

Check their understanding

'I understand that you are here regarding your child sleeping pattern and you are worried that she may have sleep-disordered breathing.'

'Firstly I would like to say that sleep disordered breathing (SDB) in children covers a variety of conditions ranging from snoring to obstructive sleep apnoea (OSA).'

'Simple snoring is not a medical problem and most children will snore at some stage of their lives. However, snoring is not only a social problem and may be associated with other significant conditions such as upper airway resistance syndrome or OSA. The latter is defined medically as recurrent events of partial or complete upper airway obstruction during sleep, resulting in disruption of normal ventilation and sleep patterns, neurocognitive deficits and cardiovascular morbidities'.

What does that mean in simple terms?

In simple terms it means that the upper airway is obstructed during sleep whilst breathing effort is still made and this can result in long term complications related to reduced intelligence and elevated blood pressure.

'My child is now 4. Will he grow out of the problem?'

In children, OSA occurs mainly between the ages of 2 and 8 years.

Earlier onset is associated with syndromes involving the head, face and nervous system eg Cruzon, Apert and Down syndrome. Later onset is related mainly to obesity.

'How do I know if my child has sleep disordered breathing?'

The diagnosis is made on taking a detailed history, with particular reference to the features to night and day symptoms such as snoring, witnessed breath holding, excessive sweating, restless sleep, unusual head position (sword swallowing position), bedwetting, frequent waking, mouth breathing, reduced oral intake, early morning headaches, mental and physical milestone delays.

Clinical examination, lateral neck x-ray (to assess the size of the upper airway) and overnight sleep study (continuous pulse oximetry) are also helpful in reaching the diagnosis.'

However, the gold standard investigation is a full sleep study called polysomnography but it is expensive and therefore reserved for syndromic children or special cases only.

'So what will treatment be if she has sleep-disordered breathing – I have heard about simple and complex surgery?'

Medical treatments consist of drugs for nasal congestion, allergies and/or acid reflux.

Continuous positive airway pressure ventilation is another non-surgical option but it is poorly tolerated in children.

In most cases the best treatment is adenotonsillectomy, which is curative.

Complex upper and lower jaw repositioning (orthognathic) surgery is reserved for children with craniofacial deformities and other complex cases.

6.15 Counsel the parent of a child with suspected otitis media with effusion (glue ear)

Brief	This mum just read about glue ear and wonder if her 4-year-old child has the condition because she has some difficulty hearing . She would like to speak to you about glue ear. Please counsel her regarding her concerns.

Introduce yourself by name and role; ask permission to speak with the patient

Check the person's relationship to the patient

Check their understanding

'I understand that you are here today to discuss the topic of glue ear. Tell me what you know and then I will answer any questions.'

'I don't know anything except that it is fluid in the ear and cause deafness.'

'Ok. Glue ear refers to the presence of (non-infective) fluid in the middle ear.'

'Why did my child get glue ear?'

The disorder arises from dysfunction of the natural tube, called Eustachian tube, which connects the ear to the back of the nose. This results in the accumulation of fluid behind the eardrum and consequently hearing loss.

Family history is a major risk factor for OME. Most children will have fluid behind the eardrums at some stage before age 11, but it usually resolves spontaneously in the majority of cases without any adverse effect. However, in some children the fluid persists and results in multiple problems related to reduced hearing, stunting of education and behavioural problems.

'How come he is not crying with the glue ear?'

Glue ear is not an infection or a painful condition. In fact, it is a silent disorder. It should not be confused with the painful red bulging eardrum (acute otitis media, AOM) associated with runny nose, fever and the upset child.

'Doctors, What are the problems associated with glue ear?'

There is strong research evidence to show that cases of persistent bilateral glue ear can result in hearing loss which in turn leads to poor speech and language development.

In addition, a history of persistent untreated glue ear is associated with a lower intelligent quotient (IQ) score, reduced reading ability and behavioural problems such as anti-social behaviour involving the law, hyperactivity, social immaturity and leaving school without qualifications.

'So how is glue ear treated? I heard a lot about alternative therapy such as homeopathy for glue ear.'

A recently published UK study (known as TARGET Trial) revealed that a period of watchful waiting for at least 3 months is beneficial as the condition may resolve spontaneously.

Medicines such as antibiotics, antihistamines or decongestants are not helpful, unless there are co-existing signs of infection or allergy.

Alternative therapies like homeopathy, cranial osteopathy, acupuncture massage and probiotics do not work. Insertions of ventilation tubes (grommets) into the ear drums have been shown to be effective, but the beneficial effect fades after 6months.

Grommets in combination with adenoidectomy (surgical removal of the adenoid at the back of the nose) prolong the overall benefits at 6-18 months. The two procedures are complementary and cost effective, especially in children with frequent upper respiratory tract infections.

In the western world, the majority of cases of chronic glue ear (greater than 3 months) are treated primarily with grommets and adenoidectomy, except in special cases such as Down syndrome where hearing aids are recommended.

'Can my child use a hearing aid?'

Yes. In non-syndromic children, hearing aids may also be used when surgery is contraindicated or not acceptable.

6.16 Counsel a parent of a child with tonsillar disease

Brief	This mum heard a lot about tonsils from her friends and wonder whether her daughter should have them removed.

Introduce yourself by name and role; ask permission to speak with the patient

Check the person's relationship to the patient

Check their understanding

'Doctor I have heard my friends speaking about tonsils. What are tonsils and what do they do?'

'The tonsils are two meatball-like lumps of tissue on either side of the back of the tongue behind the arch of the soft palate. At an early age, the tonsils help to fight infections but after that they may become less beneficial and more problematic because of size or infection. Infection of the tonsils (tonsillitis) is one of the commonest conditions in children and adolescents.

'What causes tonsillitis?'

In the majority of cases, tonsillitis is caused by a virus initially; bacteria may then become involved in the process. This is why antibiotics are often prescribed for tonsillitis, especially after 48 hours of a sore throat that is not getting better.

'So when should the tonsils be removed?'

Removing the tonsils (tonsillectomy) is a relatively common operation. Each year more than 500,000 tonsillectomies are performed in the USA, mainly because of recurrent infections or sleep-disordered breathing. In general this improves the quality of life of the patients and their family. However, not everyone with a sore throat or snoring requires tonsillectomy. The indications for tonsillectomy may be divided into **'absolute'** and '**relative**'.

Okay tell me about these indications please.

Absolute indications

In some conditions, there is no difficulty in deciding whether a tonsillectomy is required – these are referred to as 'absolute' indications; they are as follows:

1. Suspicion of cancer or metastatic head and neck cancer of unknown origin
2. Obstructive sleep apnoea secondary to huge tonsils blocking the upper airway
3. An episode of tonsillitis-associated systemic disorder such as rheumatic heart disease, kidney damage (glomerulonephritis) or chest abscess secondary to peritonsillar infection - fortunately these life threatening complications of recurrent tonsillitis are rare.

Relative indications

The 'relative' indications for tonsillectomy are debatable and the risk to benefit ratio of the procedure must be carefully considered. Essentially the argument of its opponents is that episodes of recurrent tonsillitis may represent a normal stage of development and as such are not associated with significant morbidity. If that was the case, it is logical to assume that these children would be almost equivalent to other healthy children in terms of their physical and psychological well-being, but research have shown that this is not true.

I heard my friends talking about SIGN and PARADISE. What is that all about?

In the UK and USA, there are specific guidelines to identify those who would benefit most from tonsillectomy; these criteria are commonly referred to as SIGN and Paradise Guidelines, respectively. The essence of these guideline is that tonsillectomy is beneficial if the number of episodes of tonsillitis/sore throat is:

1. At least 7 times in the previous year or
2. At least 5 times in each of the previous 2 years or
3. At least 3 times in each of the previous 3 years.

What should I do if my child gets a sore throat but not often enough to satisfy the criteria for tonsillectomy?

In such situation, other factors associated with potential significant morbidity have to be considered. These factors may be summarised as follows:

- The pattern of illness, for example, throat infections that are very severe or poorly tolerated by the child or adolescent
- Drug allergies that make antibiotic therapy difficult
- The occurrence of at least 2 peritonsillar abscesses (quinsies)
- The presence of PFAPA - Periodic Fever, Aphtous stomatitis, Pharyngitis and Adenitis (inflammation of lymph nodes).
- Febrile convulsion
- Halitosis (bad breath)
- The negative effects of recurrent tonsillitis/sore throat on the quality of life of the parents and other family members.

Other publications by the ENTTZAR TEAM

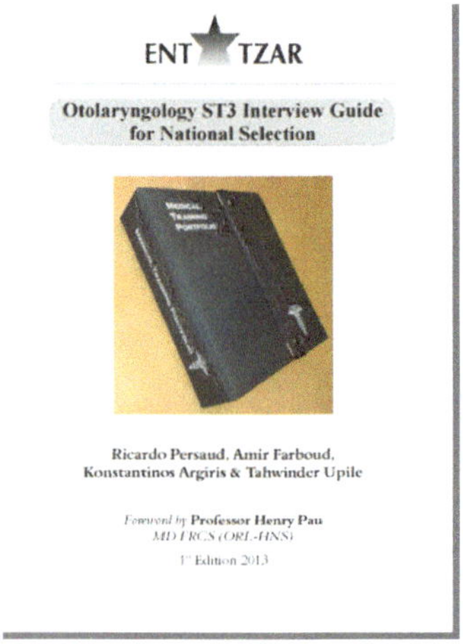

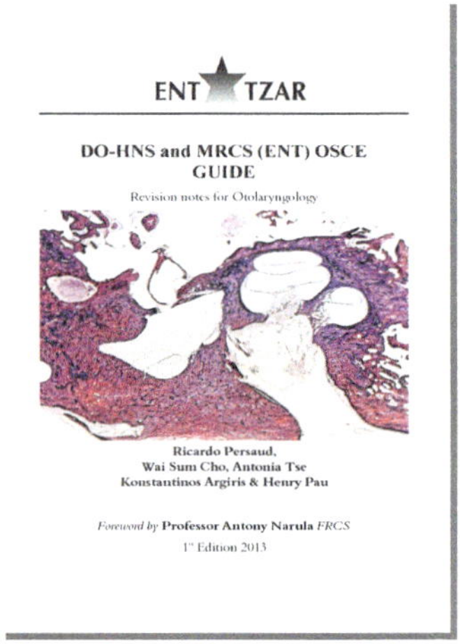

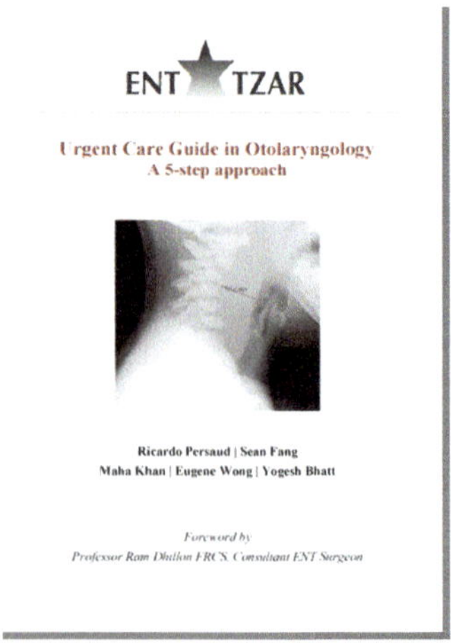

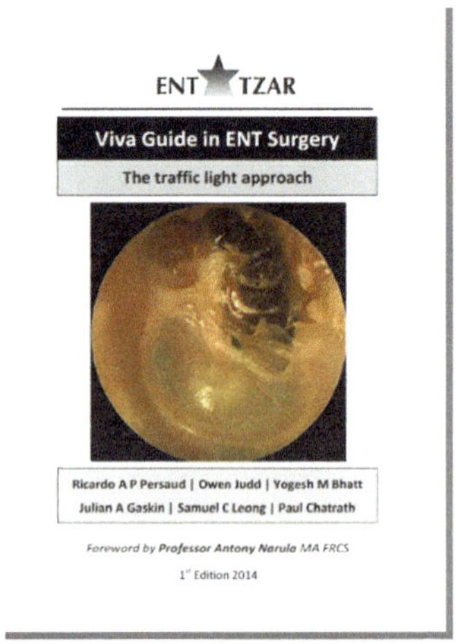

9781784561536

ND - #0114 - 050826 - C228 - 197/132/12 - PB - 9781784561536 - Gloss Lamination